The Leptin Diet

The Leptin Diet

BOARD-CERTIFIED CLINICAL NUTRITIONIST
BYRON J. RICHARDS

The Leptin Diet: How Fit Is Your Fat?

Published by Truth In Wellness Books
www.TruthInWellness.com
Tucson, Arizona, U.S.A.

Design: Design Source Creative Services

First Edition
Printed in the United States of America

ISBN: 978-1-933927-28-2

Take the Leptin Quiz at
www.WellnessResources.com

For author blog, news, and
leptin weight loss updates visit
www.TruthInWellness.com

TABLE OF CONTENTS

YOU *NEED* TO EAT. This book will explain to you *when* and *what* to eat so that you will have a much greater chance of maintaining a high quality of health over the course of your entire lifetime.

Fading from reality for many Americans is the idea of the "Golden Years," a wonderful time of relaxation, travel, enjoying grandchildren and the simple pleasures of life. How can people enjoy life and share their wisdom when they are preoccupied with crippled health?

Younger people are entering the realm of poor health at an alarming rate. Obesity, eating disorders, diabetes, asthma, and allergies now plague young Americans, creating a poor level of health that did not exist one generation ago. These problems are setting the stage for the early onset of heart disease. The handwriting is clearly on the wall.

Obesity is now one of society's major problems, the latest health epidemic. It is different than past epidemics in that there is no killer virus or bacteria to blame. In fact, it is a partly self-inflicted, slow and steady path into health oblivion. The truth is that many of us take better care of our automobiles than we do of our bodies.

When we go to the gas station we fill up the tank and stop when it is full. Indeed, our cars even have gauges that reflect true need; nobody would tolerate a broken gas gauge. We don't overfill, letting gas spill onto the streets and sidewalks, creating a public health risk. Nobody believes that we must get some gas in order to keep our engine's metabolism stoked when the gas gauge says we still have half a tank. And the idea of stopping at the gas station every time we drive by, just to top off the tank in order to be on the safe side, is not a common automotive practice. How many of us simply ignore the gas gauge altogether, stuffing ourselves and creating indigestion and heartburn? How did our society become so twisted on the subject of food?

Yes, you would like more energy and a better mood, and most likely a better body shape. If you happen to be one of the lucky, highly energized and motivated individuals with a healthy body and a drug list of zero, count your blessings. Either you are under forty, were gifted with a wonderful genetic dealing of the deck, or you have done so many things right over the course of your life that you should be awarded the gold medal of health.

Unfortunately, the human body came without an owner's manual that would give us directions about how to take care of ourselves. On a personal level this leads to considerable experimentation with ingesting food, seeking pleasure, and attempts to maintain energy and overcome stress. The results of the experiment typically leave one in a diminished state of health, sooner or later.

While it is certainly true that many factors affecting your health are under your control, the odds of your survival are stacked against you. Pollution, pesticides, and an adulterated food supply are at the top of the list.

Our food and water are contaminated to an extent that can easily disrupt the function of thyroid hormone, an issue beyond whether such pollution is carcinogenic. Virtually all people struggling with weight have functional thyroid problems, problems which seldom show up on thyroid lab tests.

The Food and Drug Administration (FDA) has officially approved chemical substances in our food supply that are so metabolically toxic it is a wonder anybody can function at all. Aspartame, used around the world to sweeten beverages, should be banned. It produces formaldehyde as it is metabolized, a fat-soluble toxin that damages hormones, the digestive tract, brain cells, or any cell membrane in the human body. Scientists feed MSG to rats in order to create and study obese rats that are not diabetic. MSG damages the subconscious brain's ability to regulate food intake, causing the gas gauge to malfunction. Why is it allowed in our food?

Even advice about what to eat is mired in vested interests and competing profit strategies. In one corner are the medical pundits preaching a low-fat and low-cholesterol diet under the guise that it will help the heart, while huge profits are reaped on the sales of cardiovascular drugs and heart operations—since this diet seldom fixes the actual health problems. In the other corner is the chicken industry, promoting the consumption of eggs while raising chickens on a diet of genetically modified organisms. Public health advice is so mired in confusion and political vested interests that we, as consumers, never know whether eating eggs is good or bad—or even if we are eating a high-quality egg.

Yes, there are many factors in our day-to-day lives beyond our personal control—factors that cause significant distress to our metabolism and contribute directly to poor health and obesity. The general public, sitting in the middle of PR campaigns from competing interests, is confused, to say the least. What is real food? How do you extract energy and health from real food?

In 2002 I wrote *Mastering Leptin*, the first book that explained to the general public the meaning of leptin and how to eat in order to be in harmony with this vital hormone. I detailed the discovery of leptin and how leptin problems cause obesity, diabetes, fibromyalgia, heart disease, and many types of cancer. Tens of thousands of people have taken advantage of this information and improved their health and metabolism by following the Leptin Diet™.

In this book I focus on the theory behind and the *Five Rules* for eating that define the Leptin Diet. Our relationship to food is strained. There are serious problems that need to be corrected. My goal is to teach you how to take charge of the hormones that control metabolism and survival. There are no recipes in this book. There is no shortage of terrific recipes readily available to one and all; I'm not trying to reinvent the wheel.

This book is the basic operating manual for how your body works in relation to food. It explains how you can extract more energy from less food, and why doing so is vital to your quality of health. This advice applies to any person of any body weight. This is not a fad approach to eating; it is what modern science has unraveled about how food actually works. While this science will continue to evolve in future years, the basic principles of its function are crystal clear and unlikely to change.

True answers for health come when people learn to properly manage their hormonal signals in relation to their challenges in life and intake of food. Healthy people eat to live, they don't live to eat. You don't have to spend the last quarter of your life limping along. You have the right to brighter future.

The human body has evolved an elaborate and sophisticated system of energy management geared for survival. You need to learn how it works. This is where we begin our journey of understanding the human body and its relationship to food and fat.

Byron Richards
October 2006

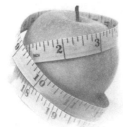

CHAPTER 1

Leptin Enables Survival

THE HUMAN BODY IS PRIMARILY CONCERNED with one thing—survival.

Fundamental to the survival of the 100 trillion cells that comprise the body is the commander in chief of operations, the human brain. On a subconscious survival level the single most important issue for the brain is energy. Food to the body, like gas to a car, is the raw material that can potentially be burned to produce energy.

The brain must make some basic calculations about energy:

1) How much and what kind of food is available?
2) How much energy will it take to acquire that food?
3) How much energy do I have to spend on various activities before I get food again?
4) Do I have enough energy to reproduce (survival of the race)?
5) Do I have enough energy to protect myself (building or finding shelter, avoiding predators, dealing with stress)?

The hard-wiring of the subconscious human brain (called the limbic system) takes these survival questions very seriously.

How is the subconscious brain supposed to know the answers? It does not have two eyes to look around and see what kind of food is available; it does not know that, in modern times, there is food on every corner. What kind of gas gauge does the subconscious brain use? How does it know when to pull over and fill up the tank?

The Discovery of Leptin

The breakthrough that provided answers to these questions occurred in 1994. For many years researchers were puzzled by a particular strain of mouse that never stopped eating. It typically became obese, diabetic, and unable to reproduce. Researchers discovered that this mouse did not make the necessary hormone to give it a *full* signal. The researchers named their newly discovered hormone *leptin*. They synthesized leptin and gave it to the mouse, at which time the animal ceased its constant eating, lost its excess weight, reversed its diabetes, and regained normal reproductive function.

This discovery set in motion one of the most intense scientific races ever—to produce a leptin drug for weight loss. Today, there are over ten thousand studies on leptin in the scientific literature. Up to this point, however, research has failed to produce any effective or FDA-approved leptin drugs. This is because only a handful of humans have the same exact genetic problem as the mouse.

Leptin Communicates to Your Brain

Leptin is made by fat cells. It travels through the blood and up to the brain. It crosses the blood-brain barrier and goes to the command center of the subconscious brain (the hypothalamus gland). The brain uses leptin as we use the gas gauge in our car. In essence, leptin in fat cells is making a phone call to the brain, informing it about how much fuel is in the gas tank.

When leptin levels are low it means that fuel reserves are running low and it's time to acquire food. When leptin levels rise during a meal it means the tank is full—stop eating. In the case of the mouse that doesn't make leptin, it never gets the *full* signal and eats itself into a disease state.

Surviving Famine

When we were evolving, the human brain could not make energy-expenditure plans based solely on one meal—simply because it did not know when the next meal was coming. It needed a way to better predict how many meals per week would be available. If enough food seemed to be coming in on a regular basis, then the body could be more permissive at "spending energy." Thus, metabolism would run faster. If, however, meals seemed scarce over a period of time, then survival instincts required metabolism to run more slowly. If too much energy was spent, the result would be starvation or perishing from malnutrition.

The brain uses leptin to perceive the amount of body fat on hand and thus gauge how much fuel has been acquired over the past several weeks. The higher the percentage of body fat, the greater the amount of leptin. Women have a naturally higher percentage of body fat, and thus higher baseline levels of leptin, because they need more energy reserves for pregnancy to enable the human race to survive. Leptin even serves an additional role during pregnancy, sustaining the growth and viability of the placenta.

During a time of abundant food and more frequent meals, the body fat of a normal-weight person will increase, compared to times of food scarcity. This fat will make leptin and that leptin level will be generally higher in the blood over a 24-hour period. This says to the brain that there is plenty of fuel on hand for long-term plans, so metabolism can be set to a higher pace. A permissive energy-spending policy can be set, since no starvation is on the horizon.

As meals become less frequent, stored fat is broken down to be used as fuel to sustain energy, which lowers the percentage of body fat. With less fat there is less leptin made over a 24-hour period. If this trend keeps up for a week or so, the brain begins to sense this general shortage of fuel and starts to tighten its energy policy, restricting metabolism.

Remember, the human body is primarily concerned with survival. During our evolution the only way to withstand a scarcity of food was to run metabolism more slowly. Once a period of starvation was over and more food was available, then depleted reserves of energy needed to be restored. There is no way one meal can restore depleted fat reserves following a longer period of starvation. Thus, as a person begins to eat more food following a period of reduced intake, the 24-hour leptin levels gradually begin to rise.

However, leptin's first task is to restore fat reserves. This is a genetic survival program. In the period of time following reduced food intake, leptin commands a large portion of calories to go directly back to fat. Gradually, over a period of days or weeks, the percentage of stored body fat is elevated, and the 24-hour level of leptin reaches a point that signifies famine is over and fat stores have been replenished. The brain, now happy with the 24-hour leptin levels, will go back to its more permissive energy-spending policy and allow metabolism to run faster.

This elegant and elaborate system is how the body spends and stores energy for survival.

The Problem of Pleasure

During human evolution there was frequently a scarcity of food, and it required considerable energy to hunt, gather, or otherwise acquire food. Thus, brain wiring developed at least ten signals that promote eating for every one signal that says to stop eating. Our brain wiring is highly tilted toward acquiring food.

Pleasure is associated with food intake. This is a survival instinct. Even when a person doesn't have a lot of energy, he or she still needs to spend energy to acquire food in order to survive. Acquiring food produces a surge of the brain neurotransmitter dopamine. This in turn produces a pleasure signal as a reward and reinforces the value of acquiring food. Mice that have no dopamine, and thus no pleasure from food intake, rapidly starve because they do not have any desire to spend energy trying to acquire food.

In contemporary life this survival principle has been turned into food addiction, which closely parallels all forms of addiction. Pain is felt in the nerves (stress, hunger, tired head), and something to produce pleasure is sought as a quick fix. Food works well. So do alcohol, drugs, cigarettes, gambling, ADHD drugs, sex, excitement, and shopping. The common theme is a substance or activity that will cause a surge of dopamine, and thus a pleasure reward for the activity. When food is used as a "solution" for stress or as a source of comfort, it typically leads to excess consumption and eventual obesity. A majority of overweight individuals are literally addicted to the taste of fat, salt, sweets, additive chemicals, and/or meals far larger than are actually needed to sustain life in a healthy way.

The Broken Gas Gauge

Unlike the mouse that makes no leptin, in humans the primary problem leading to obesity is a broken gas gauge. The gauge is stuck close to empty; thus, metabolism runs slowly even though there is an abundance of fat in storage. Unfortunately, your subconscious brain does not know what you look like in the mirror each morning. It bases your metabolic rate on its perception of leptin. If leptin is not getting into the brain, your metabolism will run slowly, a false state of perceived starvation.

This problem is called *leptin resistance*. The guidelines in this book for eating, known as the Leptin Diet, explain how to eat so that leptin gets into your brain properly. If you eat in a way that upsets the leptin applecart, you are destined for problems.

If a person cuts back a bit on junk food and excess calories, increases his or her activity or exercise, and the body then burns off the excess fat and returns to normal weight, the gas gauge is not broken. However, gaining weight through overeating and a lack of exercise places considerable stress on healthy leptin function. Once the gas gauge starts to stick, it becomes harder and harder to lose weight by reducing calories. Many overweight people find they that can eat very little and not lose weight, or that they even gain weight eating seemingly normal portions of food. Unfortunately, their gas gauge is stuck on empty. While there is still hope for fixing more difficult problems, it is much easier to fix a small leptin problem than a large one. The moral of the story: *once in shape stay in shape.*

When a person eats a moderate amount of food and maintains a reasonable amount of exercise or activity and still can't lose weight, then leptin trouble is setting in. The subconscious brain now perceives a false state of starvation, which can develop into very serious metabolic problems. When there is a broken gas gauge the subconscious brain actually thinks the current weight is the proper weight, regardless of whether the individual is twenty or a hundred pounds overweight. The brain's perception of leptin determines the set point for body weight. Tips given throughout this book will explain how to shift the set point gradually to a true normal set point and avoid inducing the starvation dieting response, which is invariably doomed to failure.

The Starvation Dieting Response

Let's take the example of a male who is twenty pounds overweight. He is not gaining weight but cannot lose weight on the amount of food he is currently eating. He begins to cut calories in an effort to lose weight. At first, his long-range metabolism is still in an energy-permissive mode, with metabolism set for the higher calorie intake.

As he cuts back on calories, metabolism runs faster for a while and he loses weight. After a week or so the drop in body fat lowers leptin levels and the subconscious brain begins to sense potential starvation. Metabolism is now reset to a slower pace to match the lower number of calories coming in. Weight loss begins to slow down or stop. At the same time, he starts to go into a starvation energy-management plan, meaning that every part of the body gets less energy. His head is now tired and irritable, muscles get weaker, he struggles with fatigue, stress tolerance is poor, and he may catch a cold or other illness because the immune system is short on energy.

Along with feeling miserable, he is no longer losing weight. If he tries to eat less he feels even worse. Typically, he is still ten pounds from a normal weight. Soon enough, he breaks down and starts eating more food. He feels better. Leptin levels begin to rise, but then the genetic program for recovery after starvation enters the picture and it says: *replenish fat.* Since the original problem of the broken gas gauge was never fixed, the brain reasons that it had better store some extra fat this time, in case the person pulls another starvation stunt. Thus all the weight is gained back, along with a few extra pounds for good measure, and only then will energy come back to something resembling normal. It could be worse: some people just keep gaining weight on a normal amount of food. They are unable to get out of the famine-recovery mode.

This is the anatomy of the yo-yo diet—survival signals gone haywire.

The Power of Leptin

Leptin is the king of hormones, the most powerful hormone in the human body. It has this lofty status because it is the commander in chief for the use of energy. The rate at which any other hormone or substance can be synthesized or function in the body requires energy, and it is leptin that gives permission to spend energy.

Science shows that leptin orders and synchronizes the behavior of all hormones. It will even micromanage when it wants to. It will take input from other hormones to help the brain figure out how to spend energy, just as the CEO of a company will take input from department heads. No other hormone orders leptin.

Furthermore, while leptin is classified as a hormone, it is structured as an immune system cytokine (messenger). And, yes, leptin is king of the immune system's function as well.

Leptin is the leader of the team, the conductor of the orchestra. It utilizes a team of hormones to carry on all energy regulation in the human body. These are powerful signals, all geared toward survival.

When a person gets on leptin's bad side, problems abound: fatigue, depression, irritability, inability to focus, poor metabolism, faulty immune function, problems extracting energy from food, high cholesterol, high blood pressure, diabetes, obesity, anorexia, reproductive-function problems—the list goes on and on. Such problems set the stage for the progression into the diseases of aging.

Learning to master leptin is the most fundamental skill required for a healthy life. It is important not just for people who are struggling with weight; it is important for everyone. Getting along with leptin helps a person to extract a maximum amount of energy from food. It is central to resolving the issue of fatigue as well as lowering all risk factors associated with heart disease. Indeed, problems with leptin are the number-one risk factor for heart disease—problems which can be set in motion in teenage years or even before.

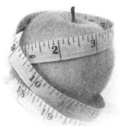

CHAPTER 2

Energy Is the Spark of Life

ALL CELLS IN THE HUMAN BODY make energy, called ATP. ATP is partly like money in your pocket, sitting there waiting to be spent. Every cell maintains a certain amount of ATP on hand, like a charged car battery. As you go into motion, existing ATP goes into action to provide immediate energy, and the cellular engines that create ATP gear up production to sustain activity.

Exercise is a way to enhance the production of ATP. Physical fitness means the body has been conditioned to produce ATP at a level of vitality. Fit individuals have more ATP at rest (well-charged batteries) and readily produce more ATP as needed (more efficient engines). Energy begets energy. It is easy to understand why couch potatoes and people in sedentary work gain weight, are fatigued, and/or struggle with mood.

People who are generally low on ATP don't have the energy to get going or the motivation to do much, like a car battery that struggles to start. They typically require some kind of jump start, like the stress of necessity or a jolt of caffeine. When unfit people get in motion, their bodies cannot sustain energy output. This results in a bad mood, fatigue, or other uncomfortable symptoms as they do things during the day. It generally means no energy to exercise, leading to even lower ATP production.

Almost everyone who exercises on a regular basis has a better mood. This is due to improved ATP function in the human body, which in turn produces more ATP so the brain can function normally.

Extracting Energy from Food

The ability to efficiently convert food into ATP is the hallmark of health. Individuals in excellent metabolic health easily extract energy from less food. The seeming need to eat a large meal in order to feel full and get some energy is a sign of inefficiency in converting food to energy. It is the start of a path toward ill health.

A *calorie* is a term used to represent the potential energy that can be extracted from food. Carbohydrates and protein have four calories per gram of food, whereas fat has nine. This means that fat, by weight, is a higher source of potential energy.

Individuals use calories differently based on a variety of factors. For example, there are people who can eat 1,200 calories a day and still gain weight or not be able to lose weight. Their ability to extract energy from food is significantly handicapped and inefficient.

By far the most common caloric problem is eating too much food. Overweight individuals are generally poisoning themselves with food. Excess sugar caramelizes and cements body structure that is supposed to be flexible. Excess fat clogs cells, organs, and arteries. Excess protein leads to nerve toxicity. While food is vital to life, too much in general or too much of any one kind is literally poison.

Hormones Are Energy Managers

The factors governing ATP production are complex. The human body has evolved a system of energy management based on substances we call *hormones*, used to orchestrate the function of one hundred trillion employees.

Hormones are made by glands in the body. They travel around and supervise the production and use of energy by cells. It is vital to understand how hormones work. Trying to understand what to eat or how to be more efficient at extracting energy from food is not possible without this knowledge.

Hormones are the energy managers, and they all answer to the boss hormone—leptin. It should come as no small surprise that leptin places a high priority on maintaining its hormonal management team, especially during times of starvation. Management is a somewhat easy task in times of abundance, ask any politician. It takes a great deal of skill to manage in times of competing needs and shortages of energy.

Thyroid Hormone—Setting the Pace

Like the drummer in the band, the body must set a tempo. This is the idling speed of the car engine. It means that at rest, or sitting at the stop sign, the body will burn a certain amount of calories in order to produce ATP. This is called *basal metabolic rate* and is governed by thyroid hormone.

Cells make energy twenty-four hours a day, seven days a week, with no vacation or overtime pay. Any time off is met with the stark reality of cellular death. Keeping cellular energy production clicking along at a pace that is based on the amount of available food is of the utmost importance to survival.

The hypothalamus gland of the brain takes input from leptin and then sets the energy spending policy for long-range plans. Leptin levels determine if enough food is present for a permissive energy plan; if so, thyroid hormone implements instructions for a higher-level idling speed.

If a person is dieting or the brain is in a false state of perceived starvation, then leptin sets a more restrictive energy-spending plan and thyroid hormone implements a conservation strategy, setting the idling speed as low as possible yet still (it is hoped) able to maintain essential functions.

Generally, this is a weekly energy management plan, since thyroid hormone made by the thyroid gland lasts 6.5 days in the blood. The body sets basal metabolic rate on a weekly basis, with an ability to slightly adjust it each day as needed. The important point to understand is that thyroid hormone does not govern acute energy needs; it guides the use of energy over a longer term, based on the supply of nutrients coming in from the diet and the general daily demands for energy facing the individual.

The classic sign that thyroid is running too slow is that an individual is cold. Normally, as cells make energy they also make heat. When the pace is too slow, not enough heat is made. In the same fashion, if a person sits down in the afternoon or evening—free of an immediate demand—and the body conks out, it is like a car stalling at a stop sign. The idling speed is too slow.

When thyroid is clicking along at the right pace it enables the use of energy for every other hormone system. There is an unmistakable feeling of being in sync.

Adrenaline—Got Horsepower?

Just as a car idling at the stop sign is not going anywhere, so it is that the human body at rest needs to step on the gas in order to get in motion, thus sending resting ATP into action. The management hormone that uses energy to implement physical action is called *adrenaline*. A single burst of adrenaline turns up energy production for two to fifteen minutes. Adrenaline is used to meet the energy requirements of changing tasks or demands as the day goes along.

Adrenaline is made in the inside part of the adrenal glands, called the *medulla*. It is also made in the nerves and referred to as *epinephrine* and *norepinephrine*. For the sake of simplicity, all three compounds will be referred to as adrenaline. An immediate cousin of adrenaline is dopamine—fundamental to reward seeking.

Most people think of adrenaline as the fight-or-flight hormone. In times of stress, adrenaline levels put the pedal to the metal so that a person can survive. Of course, this is not a good thing for people who get worked up about problems while sitting at a desk.

Adrenaline in the high-stress mode does not ask permission from cells about whether they would like to make some energy. It screams at them, forcing them into all-out action at the limits of function. *It's warp ten, Scottie!* The logic is rather simple—give it everything you've got because, if you don't, you may not be here anyway. Adrenaline can increase the metabolic ATP production in cells 600 times normal resting value (the thyroid idling speed). Such energy is not sustainable for very long, but it explains how people can perform extraordinary feats in an emergency.

In a stress-free state, adrenaline implements the use of energy for physical actions. The energy required to carry a bag of groceries in from the car requires that nerve impulses go to the muscles to coordinate the action of picking up the groceries and walking into the house. Adrenaline is what makes the muscles move and contract. Without adrenaline a person is stuck at the stop sign, idling and sputtering, or parked in bed, too tired to do anything.

There are many shades of gray between high adrenaline panic and the mundane activity of bringing in a bag of groceries. Any form of stress requires increased adrenaline output to keep up with the demands, which are typically some combination of problem-solving thought, emotional strain, and physical output of energy. The greater the demand, the greater the adrenaline required to manage the situation. Consequently, more ATP will need to be spent. Does the person have enough?

The physical weak spot for adrenaline tension is the shoulders. Too much adrenaline, compared to the ability to relax, will tighten muscles. Cramps, twitches, restless legs, and charley horses are a direct result of adrenaline stress and its wearing effect on nerves and muscles. The single common weak spot for most people is that their shoulders will tighten.

Worn-down people have frayed nerves that cannot tolerate normal adrenaline flowing through the nerves. As they try to use adrenaline, the nerves heat up, resulting in anxiety, agitation, uncomfortable sensations, a crash of energy, and eventually generalized pain in response to activity (fibromyalgia). This is the cat-on-a-hot-tin-roof problem. A person begins to feel all wound up, like a coiled spring ready to pop. True fibromyalgia is technically an allergy to one's own adrenaline, wherein adrenaline required to do normal tasks promotes an inflamma-tory immune reaction as the adrenaline travels on worn-down nerves. This problem is explained in much greater detail in the book *Mastering Leptin*.

Hormones and Behavior

Some people rely on adrenaline as a behavioral trait. The classic type-A personality is driven by adrenaline. Such people are bored by mundane work and need some sort of emergency to turn on their adrenaline engines. They will even create emergencies and conflicts where none exist, just so they have the energy to do something!

By comparison, thyroid-dominant personality types always consult because they are trying to coordinate the pace of activity. Communication, agreement, and coordinated plans are the essence of the thyroid-driven personality type. Personal strength, power, and getting the result (frequently at any cost) are the essence of the adrenaline-driven personality type. Many people use some combination of the two (a true life skill), and other people use neither strategy as a dominant type, as there are other hormone preferences influencing behavior.

Adrenaline is very compatible with testosterone, and some is required for sex drive in both sexes. Thus, when women run low on sex drive, the stress-adrenaline wear and tear has depleted them to the point where they feel no drive, and they will typically have tense shoulders as well (hint to men—back rubs are a good thing; focus on loosening up the neck and shoulder area). Women may still be able to function relatively well with no sex drive, as testosterone is not the dominant sex hormone in the female system. Once men lose sex drive it can be a serious problem, because testosterone is the essence of the survival drive in their body. In either case, low or no sex drive means declining ATP production and weakened energy-producing systems.

People Use, Manage, and Make Energy Differently

It is important to understand gland function and personality because these factors are clearly involved with how energy is used, and thus how food is acquired. Indeed, different personality types actually prefer different foods.

For example, a true thyroid personality type will not like high-fat, heavy meals. It is too much calorie-dense food coming into the body at one time, and it will literally gag the person. By comparison, the adrenaline personality type can't wait for the next high-fat, high-calorie meal. The dense, high-calorie food is the preferred fuel for kicking the adrenaline engine into high gear, whereas the thyroid type prefers a lighter meal with more complex carbohydrates and flavor. Under stress, the adrenaline type craves salt and fat; the thyroid type craves chocolate.

If a thyroid type is overweight, he or she may choose to try the high-fat, high-protein Atkins diet. But true thyroid-dominant types absolutely hate the Atkins diet; it nauseates them. It is too heavy and greasy for them to metabolize.

By comparison, adrenaline-driven type-As who have consistently consumed too much fat over the years eventually find themselves in the cardiovascular-care unit. In comes the dietician with the low-fat Dean Ornish diet, a nice diet for the thyroid personality type. Their first thought: "Where's the beef?" If they follow the Dean Ornish plan they will feel like they have been relegated to a low-energy bird-food diet that cannot possibly sustain them for any activity they are interested in doing. They may be right. On the other hand, maybe they should be happy they are still alive.

In addition to underlying personality types, there are situational "energy crises" that may cause cravings for certain types of food. A typical example is the menstrual cycle. It demands the calorie equivalent needed to perform eight hours of construction work a day for the week prior to the menstrual cycle, on top of all other energy demands for the day. A steak dinner a day of protein is put on the wall of the uterus and then discarded (not recycled) if there is no pregnancy. The menstrual cycle is about survival of the human race; thus, if there is a shortage of protein in the diet, the brain will induce signals to break down proteins from muscles and even neurotransmitters in the brain. In milder situations, as energy drops and blood sugar levels begin to fluctuate out of control, then sugar, carbohydrate, and chocolate cravings increase. If the problem is more significant, then fatty foods like ice cream, French fries, hamburgers, and potato chips are needed to offset the crashing energy.

In general, as any kind of energy crisis worsens, people will tend to crave heavy, dense food even though they may not do so on a regular basis. Some people have no appetite under heavy stress, due to the excess inflammation from the stress, which deactivates digestive function. Much more commonly, people eat in excess in order to "cool off" the feeling of stress.

Many people enter a little "energy crisis" at about four o'clock in the afternoon. Any hope they had of maintaining a good diet quickly evaporates and dooms their eating behaviors for the rest of the day. The motto of the leptin-resistant individual is, "I will start my diet tomorrow."

Maintaining Body Temperature

It is quite important to maintain internal body temperature in a range conducive to countless biological and chemical reactions that support healthy function. In general, thyroid hormone sets body temperature through the basal metabolic rate, which is adjusted gradually over time. Thyroid hormone cannot respond to a sudden drop in temperature. Leptin has figured out how to solve this problem.

The shiver response to cold is regulated by leptin activating adrenaline, which then goes to a special type of fat called *brown adipose tissue* that produces one hundred percent heat and no energy. This is a survival mechanism for cold adaptation, relevant to anyone and especially important to newborn babies so they can warm up upon entering the world.

Many weight-loss stimulants are directed at raising adrenaline to stimulate brown adipose tissue so that it disposes of calories as heat. While this manipulation has some degree of temporary success, it also depresses leptin into a starvation mode and poses considerable stress to the heart and kidneys. Once the stimulation is over, then leptin will command food to go back to storage, and weight will be regained.

New science is showing how leptin itself can act on muscles to dispose of calories as heat—a great weight-loss tool. This method is far safer, as it does not invoke starvation metabolism or stress vital organs. In essence, all one has to do is exercise.

Leptin and Adrenaline

Leptin uses adrenaline as a communication signal to fat cells, telling them to release stored fat to be used for fuel. This takes place in the course of a normal day between meals and at night during sleep. It takes place on an emergency basis anytime adrenaline is released to deal with a higher level of stress. As fat cells are broken down for use as fuel, leptin levels decline (because leptin is made by fat cells and there are now fewer fat cells). Eventually, this stimulates the desire to eat. As food is eaten, insulin levels rise, which stimulate calories to flow back to fat and increase leptin levels. As leptin levels rise, the person gets a *full* signal and quits eating. Within several hours leptin is stimulating the breakdown of fat by releasing adrenaline. This is a circle of communication, an ebb and flow between leptin and adrenaline that is based on normal meals and fuel use on a daily basis.

When a person is under stress there is an acute need for more energy. Leptin orchestrates the release of adrenaline by the brain to provide immediate energy. Not only is leptin-induced adrenaline release breaking down fat to liberate stored energy, adrenaline is also turning up the metabolic rate in the liver. Furthermore, leptin directs adrenaline straight to the kidneys to raise blood pressure so that there is enough pressure tension in the circulation to speed up the flow of all traffic on the highways of the human body. New research shows that this normal function of adrenaline under stress is actually associated with a higher level of the protective HDL cholesterol. These are all normal functions of the healthy body to deal with varying demands for energy.

Additionally, there is a synergy in the circulation between leptin and adrenaline. Over a 24-hour period there are as many as 32 leptin pulses in the circulation, an ebb and flow with adrenaline. This is a type of circulatory energy fitness, similar to the idea of muscle physical fitness. Proper pulsing between leptin and adrenaline maintains a state of readiness, so that if emergency energy systems need to be rapidly deployed, they are available.

Summary

Energy is the currency of life and metabolism. Efficiently converting food to energy is essential for good health. Without this efficiency, a person tends to overeat in an effort to gain energy from food, leading to eventual obesity and poor health.

Our bodies use hormones to manage energy. Leptin is the boss, setting energy-spending policy that is implemented by thyroid hormone. Thyroid hormone sets the pace and foundation of energy use by all cells. Adrenaline is the primary hormone that governs energy use on a minute-by-minute basis. The regulation of thyroid and adrenaline are under complex control. It is an elegant system of checks and balances, with built-in backup for emergency deployment of energy. Leptin is in charge.

People who have proper energy wake up feeling well; their energy systems turn on easily and are sustained through the day. Their head feels awake and their mood is good, even in the afternoon or evening. There is no need to eat in order to prop up energy, other than at regular meals. It is easy to take for granted the elegant system of energy management that makes all this possible, until something goes wrong. Energetic vitality is the essence of the good-health feeling.

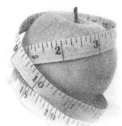

CHAPTER 3

Adapting to Demands

CAN YOUR BODY KEEP UP with the demands being placed on it?

In the previous chapter, we discussed factors that enable energy to drive metabolism, like a power boat going through the water. And like a power boat, this process leaves a wake in the water. The faster the boat travels, the larger the wake.

In human metabolism, the wake is a trail of inflammatory trash. It is how the kitchen looks after a meal has been prepared and the dirty dishes have been left in the sink.

One primary goal for a good quality of health is to produce as little inflammatory trash as possible, regardless of how fast the body is going. We all know that our car engines need oil. In the human body, the oil that keeps friction at bay is regulated by the steroid hormones produced by the adrenal glands (primarily cortisol and DHEA). Additional protection is given by the steroidal sex hormones (progesterone, estrogen, and testosterone). These are the hormones that have cholesterol as their structural backbone.

These hormones are the essence of the body's ability to tolerate stress. The adrenaline released to accomplish the activities of the day is always pro-inflammatory. This is especially true if the day is emotionally stressful or physically demanding. Other common forms of inflammatory stress include ongoing aches and pain, pollution, and infection. Additional sources—and let us all hope that we can mostly avoid them—are accidents, trauma, and intense pain.

Leptin and Inflammation

Leptin, as commander in chief, also runs the body's military—the immune system. While leptin is managing the peacetime energetic function of the human body, it does so while wearing a military uniform. In reality, new science is showing that the immune system is far more than just the military. It coordinates the entire communication and repair system of the human body.

The first phase of almost any military campaign is highly inflammatory. Leptin uses an immune signal called TNFa to carry out its inflammatory orders as well as many routine communications. TNFa stands for *Tumor Necrosis Factor alpha*, a name given to it because it will wipe out tumors if given the opportunity to do so. Like adrenaline, TNFa is an irritant that must have "oil" in order to function normally.

In addition to fighting the enemy, the immune system is involved with repair of the body. Thus, the first response to the excess demands of living is an inflammatory immune response, which is actually designed to assist repair. A highly inflammatory response is understandable in relation to an accident, injury, or illness. However, many people get a highly inflammatory response to the activities of their routine day. Some of these are from overuse, like carpel-tunnel syndrome or tennis elbow; many others are simply from the emotional or physical wear and tear of ongoing demands (a form of repetitive-strain injury). Such excess inflammation irritates the lining of the arteries and the membranes of blood cells, eventually inducing cardiovascular disease or increasing the risk of cancer.

In order to avoid getting an excessive immune-driven inflammatory response from normal living, it is necessary to orchestrate a competent anti-inflammatory response to the demands of the day. This is primarily done through the steroid hormone called *cortisol*, made by the adrenal cortex—the outer part of the adrenal glands.

Normal Cortisol

Cortisol levels are naturally highest in the morning, as they have been assigned the daily energy task of turning on all the light switches in the human body to start the day. Higher morning cortisol acts as an oil lubricant, as the engines of metabolism fire up and get going. Once metabolism is in motion, cortisol levels decline gradually during the day and reach their lowest levels during sleep (when the greatest amount of fat is being burned). This is the nonstressed daily cortisol pattern. Refreshing exercise will also elevate cortisol in conjunction with a release of beta endorphin, another potent anti-inflammatory. *Excess* exercise, however, is simply another form of wear and tear.

Stress and Cortisol

Under stress, adrenaline and cortisol rise together. Adrenaline is the irritant that increases energy output; cortisol is the lubricant that protects against the inflammation. Once adrenaline subsides, cortisol takes about sixty to ninety minutes to subside, as it is helping the body to cool off from the heat of inflammation.

Any person feeling the effects of wear and tear, poor mood, stress intolerance, sleep problems, and increasing aches or pains is now into the realm of adrenal fatigue. The adrenal glands have been working overtime, trying to keep up with the wear and tear of life. And, finally, they can't. Tolerance for stress has been depleted. The person now enters the zone of ongoing inflammation, a serious turning point in health. The hallmarks of this poor condition are no energy to exercise, feeling worse after moderate exercise, and/or persisting fatigue that is difficult to overcome. And now the immune system starts to become excessively involved in the inflammation issue, a strategy that was originally intended for acute trauma—not the ongoing daily demands of life.

Problems get worse. High cortisol and nerve inflammation, from the excess stress, keep a person awake when he or she should be sleeping—even if dead tired. Excessive cortisol ramps up the production of leptin in fat cells, contributing to surplus leptin and leptin resistance, helping to make a person gain weight. Normally, this adverse effect of cortisol on fat cells is buffered by another adrenal steroid called DHEA. However, DHEA levels drop significantly during aging or from ongoing stress, opening the door to eventual weight gain as a result of stress. Weight loss from stress is another matter entirely, and is driven by ongoing stress that results in adrenal exhaustion (the body can't make cortisol and may develop full-blown Addison's disease). Weight gain or weight loss from stress are both extremely unhealthy conditions.

The Anti-Inflammatory Team

The anti-inflammatory team comprises many factors that make up an improved ability to tolerate the demands of life. These include adequate sleep (when repair occurs), refreshing exercise (which raises anti-inflammatory endorphins—the body's natural opium), relaxing and enjoyable activities, sex, laughing, time-management and stress-management skills, among others.

The overall hormonal management of anti-inflammatory activity is carried out by the hormone cortisol, with backup support from DHEA and the sex hormones. Remember, hormones are managers—not workers. The anti-inflammatory workers on cell surfaces are fatty acids. When there is a higher omega-3 fatty acid concentration in the cell membranes, any cell has greater ability to tolerate friction and inflammation. The more a cell membrane is made up of French fries, potato chips, fried fats, trans fats, and vegetable oils, the more likely it is to become inflamed. Inside cells, the anti-inflammatory defense is based on antioxidants. As soon as a cell runs too low on antioxidants, the cell dies. End of game—no second chance.

This is why excess inflammation either causes or is a major contributing factor to all diseases of aging, essentially accelerating the onset of death. This is also why societies with diets that have a larger percentage of fresh fruit, vegetables, beans, and whole grains, compared to diets of sugar-laden processed junk, have less disease. These food are loaded with nutrients needed for basic cellular health.

Since our bodies are especially concerned with survival, the proper functioning of cortisol is vital to health. Cortisol enables the body to act like a rubber band, stretching itself in response to demands. In good health, when the stress is over, the rubber band returns to normal and the person recovers well. If there is proper elasticity in the rubber band, it can stretch and return to normal, ready to be stretched again. In poor health, the body doesn't bounce back so well, even when the stress is over. A good night's sleep isn't enough time to repair. The rubber band is losing its tone and fitness. If stress is too great, the rubber band may snap—ouch.

Having stress and responding to stress are normal parts of life. Just as the lack of exercise can make muscles unfit, the lack of stress can make the adrenals unfit. Problems occur when there is too much stress, and not enough energy is being made to enable cortisol to do its job properly.

Leptin and Cortisol

Leptin and cortisol, like leptin and adrenaline, maintain a synergistically toned relationship in health. It is part of the natural defense against stress that is orchestrated by leptin. Mice that have had their adrenal glands removed make no cortisol. These mice still have a normal leptin pattern; thus we know that cortisol does not control leptin. However, as we see in patients who make a disease level of excess cortisol (Cushing's disease), the excess cortisol ramps up excess malfunctioning leptin activity in fat cells, which causes the obesity of this disease. Thus, we know that too much cortisol helps make a person fat and contributes to leptin inefficiency.

Cortisol and Behavior

As a behavioral hormone, cortisol may produce a "high feeling" that can be relatively intense for sixty to ninety minutes. The most common example of this is the "runner's high" following exercise. It is quite intense for an hour or so and then translates to a better mood the rest of the day. On a lesser scale, a relaxed feeling from exercise comes from a small cortisol high. These are examples where cortisol is released in higher amounts than adrenaline, leaving a higher amount of cortisol in the blood relative to the adrenaline irritant.

Another time this happens is in the morning, the highest naturally occurring level for cortisol in each 24-hour period. True "morning people" have a high cortisol start to the day, similar to the runner's high feeling. In general, no one should take longer than ten to fifteen minutes to get their engines going upon awakening, although they may not feel a surplus of cortisol, as do some people. Those who find it hard to get going or are easily irritated in the morning are struggling with tired adrenal glands, not able to make enough cortisol to get the day started on the right foot. And those who run high cortisol at night, because their body is out of rhythm and dealing with too much general wear and tear, find that cortisol will cause insomnia and perpetuate fatigue the following day—a vicious circle of de-energizing poor repair.

Individuals who experience cortisol feelings at a higher-than-average level may gravitate to using cortisol as a primary behavior trait. Cortisol is a pleasure hormone; it actually hates pain. For the cortisol personality type, the driving subconscious principle is to seek pleasure and avoid pain. Such individuals will rapidly change plans or agreements based on a new possibility or something fun to do. They are the great procrastinators, experts in denial, and tend to be thrill seekers. They are always seeking the path of least resistance, with the greatest pleasure or excitement. Otherwise, pain will use up their cortisol and wreck their high feeling.

Unfortunately, eating food is one strategy for turning off

pain, a behavior called *stress eating*. This form of stress management is also employed by many people who are not dominant cortisol types; they just use the mechanism of eating food to help comfort them in order to get through the day.

High cortisol can enhance the creative function of the brain, enabling it to perceive states and relationships not possible in sequential terms. Thus, when highly creative people get into a "state," it is generally driven by a high cortisol level. This can easily become a disability if not balanced with other traits. Typical problems are ADHD, mania, and unspoken resentment— any of which may explode in a violent surge of adrenaline if cornered. An imbalanced and de-energized cortisol personality type may also display classic passive-aggressive traits.

There are considerable advantages to this personality type, especially when properly balanced with other life skills. The creative spark that powers our country is driven by cortisol. Highly talented performers, artists, journalists, architects, mechanics, construction workers, salespeople, marketers, advertisers, business trouble shooters, entrepreneurs, and many CEOs of companies all commonly have a dominant cortisol behavioral component.

When individuals learn the life skill of simultaneously combining the best traits of thyroid (planning and communication), adrenaline (the driving force to overcome obstacles and get things done), and cortisol (the creative high-power state), they are maximizing the positive use of hormonal energy to create an enjoyable and rewarding life.

When individuals get stuck in the downside of any one hormonal pattern, they are headed on a path of increased inflammation with concurrent physical dysfunction in their body. As a person starts to lose energy, any hormonal system enters into the downside of its personality traits. Behavior, hormones, ATP production, extracting energy from food, and health are completely interrelated and interdependent.

Summary

The ability to tolerate the demands of the day is essential for survival.

Ongoing anxiety and irritation, roller-coaster mood, insomnia, and a feeling of wear and tear are all signs that there are problems tolerating stress. Stress magnifies leptin problems, and weight gain is a typical result. Weight gain does not always result from stress; however, some other inflammatory problem commonly occurs.

In order to prevent disease it is vital to have a proper amount of stress tolerance in place, buffering the demands of life. Cortisol is the hormone that cools off stress, a vital function for survival. The function of this system must be maintained to the level of a well-oiled car engine. Once oil runs low, then the immune system enters a chronic low-grade inflammatory mode. This directly contributes to and speeds the onset of a poor quality of health and eventually the diseases of aging.

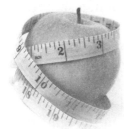

CHAPTER 4

Going to the Gas Station

ONE TASK OF THE HORMONAL ENERGY-MANAGEMENT TEAM is to solve problems in internal food distribution. As food is eaten and digested it enters into the internal working system of the human body.

The body must maintain blood sugar levels, sort fuel, store fuel, and distribute fuel. It must determine the type and quality of fuel that has been ingested and then figure out where that fuel needs to go.

Individuals who are overweight are storing more fuel than is necessary; their body is confused. The liver is the single most important organ involved in the metabolism of calories. It is the refinery where incoming food is processed, the warehouse where sugar is stored, and the distribution control center for all types of calories.

Blood Sugar

Normal fasting blood sugar contains one teaspoon of sugar for the entire gallon of blood that comprises the circulatory system. Blood is not a sweet beverage. If for some reason the body is unable to sustain this level of sugar in the blood, the brain immediately senses danger and goes into a survival mode to acquire food.

For the sake of comparison, there are six teaspoons of refined sugar in a twelve-ounce soft drink, a beverage sixty times as sweet as blood. What does the body do when the blood is flooded by sugar during the ingestion of a soft drink? Answer: *stress out*.

An ideal intake of food contains some sugar that is primarily in the form of complex carbohydrates along with fiber. Complex carbohydrates take longer to digest, thus preventing a rapid rise in blood sugar. The fiber content of the diet also slows the absorption of sugar into the blood. Even though fruit is a simple sugar, in its whole form it contains fiber that helps to slow the absorption of sugar into the blood. Fruit juice, which has been stripped of fiber, is similar to a sweetened soft drink in terms of the amount of sugar it contains and how fast it enters the system. Although fruit juice does contain nutrients of value, the effect of this much sugar on metabolism can be stressful.

It also matters if sugar is consumed on an empty stomach or as part of a meal. On an empty stomach it rushes through the stomach faster and raises blood sugar quicker. As part of a meal it sits in the stomach longer and is more slowly absorbed. Thus a banana, frequently referred to as a high glycemic index food, for its ability to raise blood sugar levels when eaten by itself, has an entirely different blood sugar reaction when consumed in conjunction with fat, fiber, and/or protein. Thus, blending a banana into a protein drink in the morning makes a great breakfast that helps to sustain proper blood sugar levels during the day.

In addition to the kind of sugar influencing blood sugar levels, the size of a meal also matters. The larger the meal, regardless of the type of food eaten, the higher the rise in blood sugar during the digestive process that takes place over the next several hours.

How Blood Sugar Is Controlled

The intake of food triggers the release of the hormone insulin by the pancreas. The larger the meal, the higher it is in refined sugar, and the lower it is in fiber, the greater the rise in insulin, because insulin is the hormone that transports sugar out of the blood. Beyond the small amount of sugar needed in the bloodstream to maintain energetic function, insulin manages the flow of calories out of the blood and to a location that hopefully wants them. It is vital to understand that insulin promotes storage of calories, the opposite of fat burning.

Following a meal, insulin wants to place about forty percent of extra calories in muscles, so the muscles have an available reserve of sugar should they need to quickly use energy. Of course, your muscles only need sugar if you have been active and have used some of the existing sugar already stored. This is why a consistent exercise program and physical activity are vital for the fitness of the insulin transport system.

The other place insulin would like to store sugar is your liver. The liver is the primary warehouse and distribution center for calories. Insulin will deposit approximately sixty percent of the calories in your liver, if it can. This will only happen if the liver actually needs them, which will be discussed shortly.

If the muscles and liver don't want sugar, then sugar is transferred to fat. It is packaged up into triglycerides and then sent to the stomach, hips, thighs, or generally distributed to various areas to increase the existing amount of fat mass.

Triglycerides are how the body stores fuel in a compact and efficient manner. Each triglyceride is composed of one sugar and three fatty acids. Some triglycerides are present in the blood, as an accessible source of energy, should you need them. The fat cells in white adipose tissue are filled with triglycerides. This is normal. If you are trying to lose weight, you are seeking to find a strategy that will cause triglycerides to be released from your fat cells. Once released, they must be broken down into their individual pieces (one sugar and three fatty acids), which can then be used by cells as fuel. If you are gaining weight, your body is storing too many triglycerides.

Insulin directly promotes the formation of triglycerides. It is not technically possible to break down stored fat, and thus lose weight, during an insulin-dominant time. This is because insulin promotes storage. An insulin-dominant time is anytime a person eats; and depending on the quantity of food just eaten, the insulin dominant time generally lasts three to four hours.

Insulin and Leptin

A drop in leptin signals hunger. Food intake stimulates insulin release. As a person eats, insulin is always directing some amount of triglycerides to go over to white adipose tissue and enter fat cells. This is normal. It is a form of communication that tells the white adipose tissue that food is being acquired. This turns on the production of leptin in fat cells, causing the blood level of leptin to rise in response to the meal. As the leptin levels rise high enough, they signal to the brain that enough food has been eaten. Leptin now signals the pancreas to stop making insulin. There are many leptin receptors in the pancreas. Properly functioning leptin in a healthy individual appropriately turns off the production of insulin, as well as providing a proper *full* signal to the brain.

In overweight people, the communications involving insulin and leptin are inefficient. It is like making a phone call where no one answers. Insulin resistance and leptin resistance mean that the hormones don't communicate efficiently in response to food. Thus a person has to overeat in order to get enough leptin into the brain to get a *full* signal. The pancreas may not hear the leptin signal to stop making insulin, which leads to excess insulin, fatigue, and possibly even more hunger within a few hours of eating. This can also lead to a drop in blood sugar three or so hours after eating, because blood sugar management hormones are stressed out and have a hard time doing their job. Several hours following the meal the extra insulin ends up taking too much sugar out of the blood, making a person hungry and tired-headed.

What Is Normal?

The advice to eat five to six small meals a day or to snack between meals to maintain a steady blood sugar level and keep metabolism "stoked with food" is among the worst advice possible. It boggles the mind that a majority of doctors, dieticians, nutritionists, and fitness instructors promote this absurd approach to energy management. It is as if someone started a bad rumor and everyone accepted it as a truth.

If a person does lose weight eating this way, it is usually because he or she is eating fewer calories in total than before. This may "work" for a few weeks, until leptin levels readjust to the new level of calorie intake and slow down metabolism. However, this eating strategy inhibits normal fat burning by interfering with the proper function of leptin and insulin.

These are the simple facts that will never change: Eating food raises insulin. Insulin promotes storage of calories and prevents the burning of stored fat for fuel.

How to Burn Fat

Three to four hours after a meal, blood sugar levels naturally begin to drop because insulin has done its job of transporting calories about the body. Now it is time to use stored calories. The drop in insulin signals the pancreas to produce another hormone, called *glucagon*. Glucagon's job is to maintain the blood sugar level in the absence of food coming in from the diet. This is normal.

Glucagon goes over to the liver and knocks on the liver's door. It says, "You stored sixty percent of the calories following the last meal. I need some of those to maintain blood sugar levels." Glucagon is the manager, the liver obeys orders. The liver now converts stored sugar (glycogen) back into blood glucose to maintain blood sugar levels.

Yes, the body is getting a "snack." Instead of coming from food, the meal comes from sugar stored in the liver. This is liver fitness and normal function. Between meals, about sixty percent of fuel will now be sugar coming from the liver. In the flame of burning sugar, and under the influence of glucagon, the liver will now burn forty percent fatty acids. Triglycerides are now broken down to be used as fuel. This starts happening three to four hours after a meal and continues until the next meal is eaten. This is a fat-burning time.

The longer a person is in this fat-burning mode, the greater the amount of fat he or she will burn—as long as energy level is maintained. A healthy person who has not eaten for four to five hours prior to bed will burn sixty percent fatty acids and forty percent sugar the last three to four hours of sleep, a prime fat-burning time. If a person eats before bed it shuts off this prime fat-burning time during sleep.

If a person eats a snack it raises insulin and shuts off fat burning. Even worse, the liver never uses any of its stored sugar. Because this sugar was never used, calories eaten at the snack now can't go into the liver as part of the normal storage function of insulin. Instead, the calories are headed in the direction of fat formation, even if the snack contained no fat grams.

Snacking flips on the insulin switch at the wrong time, which causes the consumed calories to head for fat storage. This is true even if a snack contains only fifty to a hundred calories. Anything that was a fatty acid headed for energy production is now repackaged as a triglyceride and stored: *fat burning stops*. This is why snacking and eating five to six meals a day is such a bad idea. Those perpetuating this way of eating as a means to stabilize blood sugar are actually fueling insulin resistance and leptin resistance. In reality, this significantly contributes to the societal epidemics of obesity and diabetes, inducing metabolism to function in a crippled manner. Snacking or eating too often confuses leptin, and sooner or later this catches up with an individual.

Summary

Up to this point I have explained three major roles of hormones in relation to energy management and food intake: 1) driving metabolic action, 2) adapting to the demands of stress, and 3) distributing and transporting fuel. These hormonal activities all have one basic purpose—survival.

Hormones are energy managers. Understanding them and

eating so as to facilitate their functions in the body is essential to health. Now that you understand how these hormones work, it will be much easier to understand why eating a particular way can make such a difference to your health.

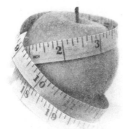

CHAPTER 5

The Five Rules of the Leptin Diet

Do you remember the last time you popped out of bed in the morning bright-eyed, bushy-tailed, and ready to go? Your energy was good all day long. You felt in rhythm, like you were clicking along to the beat of your own goals. You had the energy to deal with the challenges of life. You were in charge. Symptoms of your body were not a distraction, and you maintained normal body weight without too much effort. Your body was a tool that was grounded in the subjective feeling of vitality. Your enthusiasm, motivation, and spark for living were an example and inspiration to others. And at the end of the day, normal tiredness assisted you into an undisturbed and rejuvenating sleep. You woke the next morning to find yourself once again ready to tackle life.

This paragraph describes a person with normal energy. If you don't feel this way, don't try to rationalize why you don't. Aging is a wonderful excuse; there are many others. They hold no validity in the eyes of leptin. Leptin wants normal energy so that you can survive. As a side effect you will have a great quality of health.

In order to get normal energy you must extract it from food. This means that you should seek to eat in harmony with leptin. Doing so enables your hormonal energy managers to function with the fewest challenges. Yes, you can eat other ways. And, minimally, it will be like rowing a boat against the current. Eat smart, be smart. When you use less energy to digest food, transport food, and deploy food into action, you will have more energy left over for activities of your choosing.

Successfully Managing a Complex Operation

It is amazing to realize the elegant complexity of leptin's executive skills in overseeing the operation of more than one hundred trillion energy-producing employees. Behind every great CEO is a great management team, and leptin's team is nothing short of spectacular. All great managers make things simple. Thus, it is not surprising that you need only follow five easy rules to eat in harmony with leptin.

No set of rules can cover every health variable. Some conditions and exceptions apply here and there and are worth knowing about. However, these five simple rules form the essence of how to extract more energy from less food. Following them readily supports a higher quality of health, enables metabolism to run better, and helps prevent poor health in older years. These rules form the core eating plan of the Leptin Diet.

The Leptin Diet is based on fundamental scientific truth. The principles upon which it is based are unlikely to change. This is not a fad diet, a calorie-manipulation scheme, or a starvation routine masquerading as a diet. It does not involve deprivation of pleasure. While the emphasis of this book may seem directed at those who need to lose weight, the underlying principles of the Leptin Diet apply to most people. It is a lifestyle for eating properly, grounded in the science of leptin. It is something you can do happily and healthfully every day for the rest of your life. The diet is energizing!

The *Five Rules*

The Leptin Diet consists of five key dietary rules, called the *Five Rules*.

Rule 1: Never eat after dinner. Allow eleven to twelve hours between dinner and breakfast. Never go to bed on a full stomach. Finish eating dinner at least three hours before bed.

Rule 2: Eat three meals a day. Allow five to six hours between meals. Do not snack.

Rule 3: Do not eat large meals. If you are overweight, always try to finish a meal when you are slightly less than full: the *full* signal will usually catch up to you in ten to twenty minutes. Eating slowly is important.

Rule 4: Eat a breakfast containing protein.

Rule 5: Reduce the amount of carbohydrates you eat.

The first three rules form the core of the Leptin Diet. Rule 4 is important for anyone trying to lose weight or overcome fatigue. Rule 5 is included because most people struggling with weight eat too many carbohydrates, and it serves as a reminder of how important it is not to do so.

Rule 1: Never eat after dinner.

One of leptin's main rhythms follows a 24-hour pattern. In this pattern leptin levels are highest in the evening hours and peak late at night. This is because leptin, like the conductor in the orchestra, sets the timing for nighttime repair. It coordinates the function of melatonin, thyroid hormone, growth hormone, sex hormones, and immune system function to carry out rejuvenating sleep. It does this while burning fat at a greater rate than at any other time of the day. And it accomplishes this only if you allow it to do so.

In a person who is developing or who possesses normal leptin function, the naturally higher level of leptin in the evening hours enters into the brain and says: "You are not hungry and your energy systems are running in an energy-permissive mode—meaning you feel good." You may be energetically wind-ing down from a busy day, but there is no abnormal tiredness, grumpiness, or craving for food.

By comparison, those with leptin problems assume a differ-ent personality type in the way they eat after four o'clock in the afternoon. They are stuck in the problem of leptin resistance. Leptin levels may be high in their blood, but leptin is not get-ting into their brain. Thus they never get a proper *full* signal (until they overeat) and they are driven by subconscious urges to acquire food—urges that are far greater than willpower and self-discipline can manage.

Dinner is over and eating begins. They circle the refrigera-tor and the kitchen cupboards, like an animal hunting its prey. They frequently find any excuse to obtain food, in the house or out of the house. Or they plop themselves in front of the TV and begin to eat, their reward for all they have been through that day. They are living in the leptin nightmare, driven to ac-quire food even though rationally they know they don't need it. They don't understand why the mere idea of eating their favor-ite foods causes them to salivate. Was Pavlov really right?

Finally, they end the evening with a nice bowl of ice cream. Having eaten themselves into a condition of abnormal fatigue, their appetite is now finally satisfied and they are ready for bed, and a rotten night's sleep. They will burn no fat from their hips, thighs, or stomach—they will add to the existing mass. And, yes, they will get up the next morning feeling crummy and pledge themselves to a better day—waiting for the battle with misdi-rected leptin later that evening, a battle they will never win.

It is easy for me to tell you not to eat anything after dinner. So I am going to do so. In order to get back on track, the first thing you need to know is what you are supposed to be doing. If you have a lighter dinner, wait at least three hours before going to bed. If dinner is your largest meal of the day, allow five to six hours between the time you finish eating and the time you go to bed. If you don't think this rule fits your lifestyle, think again.

Rule 2: Eat three meals a day.

Another rhythm of leptin involves its regulation of the *full* signal in relationship to a meal. In order to avoid nighttime leptin problems it is necessary to manage leptin properly during the day. Poorly managed leptin during the day sets the stage for the disaster experienced at night.

Leptin and insulin work together to ensure meal adequacy and the ability of the body to transport the calories ingested to various locations in the body that need them. There is no such thing as a diet that creates no rise in insulin after a meal. Insulin rises in response to food intake because it has an important chore to perform. Once this process is over, a person can now enter a true fat-burning mode.

It is vital to create times during the day when triglycerides are cleared from the blood. If triglycerides build up during the day, they physically impede the entry of leptin into the brain, causing leptin resistance. Our evolutionary metabolism is not designed to deal with constant eating and snacking. When a person eats a snack it raises insulin, shuts off fat-burning mode, and allows triglyceride levels to stay too high for proper leptin function—reducing proper leptin entry into the brain. In turn, this causes excessive food cravings, an unstable energy level, poor head function, and unproductive sleep. Snacking sets off a domino effect in metabolism that is devastating to health. Ingesting food flips powerful hormonal switches—quite a different notion of diet than one that simply counts the calories we eat.

It is fine if a person wants to eat fewer than three meals a day, as long as energetic function is properly maintained and there are adequate calories in the diet. Many people who sleep in on the weekend will find that a larger brunch-type breakfast along with dinner are all they need. In this way they will have no trouble maintaining the proper number of hours between meals.

When individuals do a good job of managing leptin during the day, blood levels of triglycerides are not piled up and backlogged. Now, when they go to sleep, they will enter fat-burning mode. As the night moves on, healthy people will end up burning sixty percent fatty acids during sleep, the prime fat-burning time. People who manage leptin well will burn fatty acids coming from the triglycerides that are stored in the abdominal area, hips, and thighs. This is the secret to successfully losing weight and maintaining a healthy weight. People who are struggling with leptin tend to burn fatty acids during sleep from triglycerides that are piled up too high in the blood, due to all the eating mistakes of the day.

Rule 3: Do not eat large meals.

The fastest way to cause leptin problems is to eat large meals. It does not matter whether a meal is composed mostly of fat, carbohydrate, or protein. Large meals are the easiest way to poison the body with food.

Unfortunately, portion sizes in today's world are too large. Individuals tend to eat whatever is in front of them. If a super-sized portion is ordered, served, or available as a second serving, a super-sized portion will be eaten. This problem is made worse by the simple fact that individuals with leptin problems cannot get a proper *full* signal from an adequate amount of food. In fact, they may not get a *full* signal for perhaps a half hour after they have eaten a sufficient amount of food. Even worse, if there is any food still available to eat, leptin-resistant people tend to go past any *full* signal they do get.

The leptin-resistant person subconsciously defines a *full* signal based on two points: 1) consumption of anything in sight, and 2) feeling stuffed.

Anything short of this leaves them with a nagging feeling of deprivation or dissatisfaction. These individuals know that if they just eat enough they will feel so much better. True enough, when they hit their satisfaction point they do feel better and are in a better mood. The problem is that they are speeding the onset of poor health with the excess calories they mistakenly thought they had to eat.

The ready availability of food and the large portions commonly offered play into this disease-producing pattern of consumption. No leptin-driven food addict will order a salad and lean protein when salivating for a high-fat, high-calorie meal. All makers of fast food know it: their profits are based on it. It is totally ridiculous that these companies portray themselves as doing public health a favor by offering "lighter" versions on their menus. Their menus contribute in a big way to our society's obesity epidemic and poor quality of health. They market directly to the subconscious problems of a society full of food addicts—a situation they helped to create in the first place.

The number of calories that should comprise a meal varies based on a person's physical size, activity level, and any needed weight loss. The daily calorie need for women generally falls somewhere in the 1,200 to 1,800 calorie range; for men the range is somewhere between 1,600 to 2,200 calories. Sedentary individuals fall on the lower side of this range; moderately active people on the higher end of this range. These are general guidelines. Intense physical activity requires higher caloric intake.

A person does not need to divide calories equally among meals. A larger lunch helps most people get through the afternoon. Arriving home for dinner ravenously hungry and tired is almost certain to result in overeating.

Rule 4: Eat a breakfast containing protein.

A high-protein meal can increase metabolism by thirty percent for as long as twelve hours—the calorie-burning equivalent of a two- to three-mile jog. A high-carbohydrate breakfast such as juice, cereal, waffles, pancakes, or bagels does not enhance metabolic rate by more than four percent, especially when eaten with little protein.

This rule is especially important for individuals who struggle with energy, food cravings, and/or body weight. In general, Rule 4 is a necessity for anyone over the age of forty. While some people may be able to run their metabolism just fine on a higher carbohydrate breakfast for a number of years, this tends not to be the case once any type of metabolic problem sets in.

Higher protein meals that are not too large help to reduce the amount of insulin released, as well as enhance the release of glucagon when it is needed to sustain energy between meals. Since these are major problems in a leptin-resistant individual, starting the day off on the right foot is a very good idea. A glass of fresh juice in the morning, healthy as it may seem, is likely to flare up leptin problems later in the day.

The two signs of a poor breakfast are: 1) being unable to make it five hours to lunch without food cravings or a crash in energy; and, 2) being much more prone to leptin resistance later that afternoon or evening, a condition that sets in motion strong food cravings.

Eggs are a good breakfast, just not smothered in butter and cheese. Cottage cheese is another high-protein breakfast food, and along with a serving of complex carbohydrate or fruit, it makes a great breakfast. Even a few tablespoons of peanut butter or almond butter (not half the jar) on a piece of toast may be adequate, especially if a person is in a hurry. Whey protein smoothies are another easy way to start the day. Any lean protein can be eaten at breakfast, along with a moderate amount of carbohydrates and a reasonable amount of fat.

Rule 5: Reduce the amount of carbohydrates you eat.

Carbohydrates are easy-to-use fuels. The body takes "money" from its wallet—the food on a plate—before it dips into the savings account: the hips, thighs, buttocks, and midsection. Carbohydrates in the diet are the main signal for insulin secretion. If there is a problem with insulin resistance and leptin resistance, as is the case with most overweight individuals, then cutting back on carbohydrates helps reduce these problems.

Some carbohydrates are needed in a healthy diet. Too few carbohydrates may cause thyroid hormone malfunction, electrolyte disturbances, muscle weakness, depressed release of growth hormone, poor fat burning, an unsatisfied feeling after a meal, cardiovascular distress, and poor digestion.

Individuals who go on the Atkins diet frequently become car-bohydrate cripples. They train their bodies into carbohydrate inefficiency, which is worse than their original problem of simply eating too many carbohydrates. Now, when carbohydrates are eaten, they turn on the weight-gain switch. A healthy diet that promotes weight loss should include all types of calories.

In general, many overweight individuals eat two or more times the amount of carbohydrates they are able to metabolize. When carbohydrates are reduced, fat or protein in the diet need to increase so that there are enough calories to function. Finding the right balance takes time and paying attention to your body. Every meal of the day does not have to be the same. The goal is to be able to go five to six hours between meals with a good energy level and to lose weight or maintain proper body weight.

In most cases, just getting the protein and carbohydrates into better balance goes a long way toward promoting weight loss. This is easily done with the visual fifty-fifty technique. Look at meals and see a palm-size piece of protein (a four- to six-ounce portion for women; six- to eight-ounce portion for men). When trying to lose weight, keep the total carbohydrate physical size the same physical size as the protein, a fifty-fifty visual. This way, there is no calorie counting. Compare the protein (chicken, meat, turkey, eggs) to the carbohydrates (bread, rice, pasta, potatoes, fruit, corn, squash, etc,). Fill up on fiber-rich vegetables as desired.

If dessert is on the menu, plan to skip most of the carbohydrates in the meal. Instead, have a large salad or extra vegetables with the protein serving. If carbohydrates are eaten during the meal, then take only one or two bites of dessert.

Summary

The *Five Rules* of the Leptin Diet are designed to enhance the function of hormones that regulate the production of energy. This, for some, is not a new or revolutionary way to eat. What is new about this is *why* you need to eat this way.

Remember one key message about the science of leptin: *When* you eat is just as important as *what* you eat. Eating throws powerful hormonal switches. Make sure you throw them at the right time so that your body can do what it was intended to do. Eating in harmony with leptin will make your life easier.

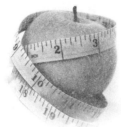

CHAPTER 6

Adjusting to Your Meals

THE *FIVE RULES* FORM THE CORE SYSTEM for eating in harmony with leptin. A literal interpretation of the rules means that a person gets up in the morning and has breakfast, eats lunch five to six hours later, and eats dinner five to six hours after that. In a perfect world this plan is quite workable. In the hustle and bustle of everyday life, sticking to such a plan is sometimes hard. Scheduling may require various adjustments in the rules.

Another common problem for some people is the seeming inability to follow the rules without experiencing troubling symptoms. When people have low blood-sugar symptoms between meals, they may become jittery, get a headache, or feel their energy level crash. Does this mean the *Five Rules* are flawed? No; the inability to follow the *Five Rules* reflects a poor level of metabolic physical fitness. Just as most people would agree that going for a three-mile jog is good exercise, many people are hard pressed to run even a block or two. Does that mean jogging is bad?

Not everyone is fit enough to follow the *Five Rules* at first. They may need to build up to them. Some people find it hard to believe they could ever go five to six hours without eating, but a few days of willpower will get them out of the seemingly desperate clutches of faulty leptin-driven cravings and into metabolic gear. Much to their surprise, following the *Five Rules* is not only easy, but energy level increases and numerous other troubling symptoms magically begin to disappear. This is by far the most common response to following the *Five Rules*.

Plan Your Day

Breakfast is important. If you have only four hours until lunch then you need a lighter breakfast (300 to 400 calories). If you have five to six hours until lunch, you need an average-size breakfast (450 to 550 calories).

If you have a heavy exercise workout scheduled that morning (or have already exercised intensely before breakfast), a demanding physical job, or you have to go six or seven hours until lunch, eat a larger breakfast. If you get up late or don't have time to eat first thing, then your breakfast time is sliding into a brunch time. Unless you eat three light meals, you are now on a two-meal-a-day plan and need a larger meal that will last you seven hours until dinner (600 to 700 calories).

The goal is to get at least 20 grams of protein at breakfast, and at least 30 grams if breakfast is a larger meal. Some individuals will function much better on 40 to 50 grams of protein at breakfast. The goal of a good breakfast is to get a stable base of protein and an appropriate amount of calories to sustain your energy needs so that you can make it to your next meal without needing to eat. A good breakfast and a stable morning period also lend stability to the afternoon and evening "weak spots" that are the metabolic downfall of many individuals.

If you don't know the calorie content of the foods you are eating or how many grams of protein they contain, then go online and type in "calories" in your browser. There are many websites offering easy-to-use calculators that show not only the calories of all common foods, but also their grams of protein, fat, and carbohydrates.

The idea of planning a good breakfast is not to become obsessed with calorie counting, but to have an understanding of portions of food you like to eat—portions that will hit a certain calorie range and provide adequate protein for metabolic support. Many individuals may be surprised that foods they thought were bad for their health actually provide great energy and are terrific support for metabolism, when eaten in the proper amounts. Saturated fat is a very easy to use fuel that can significantly support healthy liver function to help maintain a good energy level. It is only when a person eats too much saturated fat and combines it with large amounts of refined sugar and refined grain that it becomes a health risk, as there are simply too many calories to use.

Breakfast

The following breakfast qualifies as a "light meal," even though you might not think so at first glance:

	Calories	Grams of Protein
2 poached or hardboiled eggs	150	12
1 slice of Canadian bacon	68	9
1 slice of whole grain toast	65	2
1 tab of butter	27	0
Coffee with 1 tablespoon cream	52	0
Total	362	23

Other examples:		
8 ounces of 2% cottage cheese	203	31
1 cup of fresh fruit	50-80	1
1 slice of whole grain toast	65	2
Total	318-348	34

Blend the following:		
1 scoop whey protein	110	24
1 medium banana	100	1
8 ounces 2% milk	120	8
Total	330	33

Real food is always good for you when it is eaten in the right amounts. When we eat too much food our hormonal energy managers get in a funk, causing us to produce less energy even though we are eating more. By eating real food in harmony with your hormonal management team, you can extract more energy from less food.

Don't be brainwashed by campaigns that portray saturated fat and cholesterol as evil. These have turned our society into paranoid food consumers. There is nothing worse than a recipe book full of egg dishes made with egg whites. What a joke.

A majority of people cannot sustain metabolic energy on a low-fat diet. This is not simply my opinion. Test it for yourself. There are not many people who will feel metabolically normal when less than thirty percent of their total calories come from fat. Low-fat diets are not the answer to weight loss, maintaining normal body weight, or preventing heart disease.

There are many breakfast options and many recipes for all kinds of breakfasts readily available on the internet or in numerous publications. Try to get at least 20 grams of protein at breakfast and realize that you, personally, may feel much better eating up to 50 grams of protein at this meal. Pay attention: Need varies greatly based on individual metabolism, activity level, and stress. The key is not to be found in a specific number of grams of protein, but rather in starting the day on the right foot, which will result in a more stable metabolism.

Lunch

The goal of lunch is to eat the right amount of food so that you can make it to dinner without crashing during the afternoon. Many individuals eat a skimpy lunch, thinking they are doing a great job of dieting. By the middle of the afternoon they are circling junk-food machines or rapidly plummeting into the depths of leptin despair, knowing they will not be able to control their eating pattern the rest of the day.

Many people do better eating a larger lunch and a smaller dinner. This is difficult if the family gathers at dinner, which often makes dinner the largest meal. However, the goal is to eat enough at lunch so that one is not arriving home ravenously hungry and/or tired.

The easiest way to go longer between any two meals is to add some fat to the first meal. A few ounces of cheese or nuts added to a basic lunch will typically enable a person to have better energy through the afternoon. Another remedy is to try to push lunchtime back so that there is less time until dinner.

When leptin, hormonal systems, and food are working well, then a person will maintain good energy throughout the afternoon and arrive at dinner with a normal appetite that is under control. One noticeable sign of how well these systems are working is how one's head feels in the late afternoon. A tired, grumpy, heavy, or irritable head are signs that things are not going so well and metabolism is about to have a power outage. A metabolically fit person eats breakfast and lunch in the right amounts of food to sustain energy between meals. No snacking is needed.

Dinner

Getting home late, eating the largest meal of the day, and then going to bed is a fast way to cause leptin problems. Always allow three hours before bed following a light dinner (300 to 400 calories). If dinner contains 600 calories or more, allow at least five hours until bedtime. This spacing is vital for proper metabolism.

Individuals prone to insomnia should eat their main proteins of the day at breakfast and lunch. Dinner should be higher in complex carbohydrates. Some people need protein at every meal to keep their metabolism running normally; others simply need a noticeable protein serving at two of their three meals. A 6-ounce portion of fish, chicken, or red meat averages 40 to 50 grams of protein per serving. Moderately active people typically need half their ideal body weight in grams of protein per day. Some need more and some need less; this is a general rule of thumb.

Because protein activates the metabolism, individuals who eat too much protein at dinner, or who eat more total protein in a day than they really need, may find themselves unable to fall asleep. Eating more complex carbohydrates in the evening meal with lower protein helps to elevate the amino acid tryptophan, which in turn promotes melatonin release and an easier time falling asleep.

Too much protein can induce a toxic reaction, a condition of excess ammonia and excess excitation of brain neurotransmitters. This type of reaction is not energetic. The symptoms are tiredness within a half hour of eating, a heavy or irritable head, and/or a headache. It is easy to identify whether the amount of consumed protein is the problem. Simply eat a smaller amount of protein and see if these symptoms still occur within a half hour of the meal.

This problem is most common for individuals trying to eat a high-protein and low-carbohydrate or low-fat diet. Sometimes just adding some carbohydrate or fat will prevent the large spike of protein into the brain following a meal. A protein drink in water, with no other food, is not typically a good idea. Every calorie type is vital to life, in the proper amount. The Leptin Diet advocates a solid base of protein to fortify energy stability through the day, always eaten in combination with other types of calories.

The Dinner Preparation Problem

Dinner is a difficult time for individuals wrestling with leptin. The leptin-resistant chef starts in with "nibble time," otherwise known as meal preparation. This chef, either due to subconscious cravings, the complaints of a spouse with out-of-control leptin urges, and/or the real need to feed growing children, tends to lose track of portion size. Enough food is prepared to feed an army. Not only is the first serving too large, there are second servings as well. A child who is of normal body weight, physically active, and growing may be able to utilize those calories. Everyone else struggles.

Overweight individuals need at most a 6-ounce portion of protein per meal. If you are trying to lose weight, try to keep your total "pleasure" carbohydrates in the range of 200 to 300 calories. Add up any calories in beverages, bread, pasta, grains, potatoes, corn, squash, rice, fruit, and dessert and figure out what you really want to eat. Eat as many vegetables as you want. Salad dressing is a big factor in the total calorie count of any meal, frequently making salad as bad as pizza. You don't want to live as a calorie counter; however, ignorance of the calorie content of food is far worse. Know the calories in food well enough to be able to plan appropriate portions.

Plan all portions before the meal and put away any extra food before the meal starts, while your conscious brain still has some semblance of control. For most people, this strategy means that dessert is bite size, if any is eaten at all. Learn to share. Choose the flavors you want from real food, but don't exceed your portion. Slow down, make conversation. A relaxing dinner should last at least a half hour. And ideally a meal is completed within one hour from start to finish. Pace your food, enjoy your dinnertime.

Realize that the urge of leptin is to eat until you are satisfied. The big problem is that "satisfied" for a leptin-resistant person is not based on a needed or normal amount of food. A correct *full* signal from a normal amount of food may take a half hour to reach the brain in this seemingly deprived individual.

Plan activities after dinner and get onto them. Such activities should never allow access to food. The buddy system really helps. Perhaps spend more time with your spouse doing fun things together, helping each other stay on track. Find a new activity. Do anything! Sitting on the couch in front of the TV is only a few short steps from the refrigerator; too close to win a battle with out-of-control leptin. Get busy.

The *full* signal will catch up soon enough and you will be surprised that you feel satisfied and "energized," even though you didn't eat more. Leptin has now given permission for your metabolism to run. As you improve, this is how you will feel immediately after a normal-size meal.

Until you have a well-established pattern of normal portion intake, and the *Five Rules* are truly a way of life, it is best to have some kind of buddy system at night. Leptin problems can be worse than any drug addiction and are especially difficult to overcome for people with a history of drug or alcohol abuse. As you lie down to go to sleep at night, having successfully made it through the leptin bewitching hours, a glimmer of hope begins to shine through the darkness of the leptin clouds. Standing on the scale the next morning, hope is typically fortified by encouraging results.

Exercise

Exercise at any time is better than no exercise. Any exercise helps condition muscles to use fuel and helps strengthen the liver's ability to manage the flow of calories. Consistency in an exercise routine is of the utmost importance. Long walks, forty-five minutes to an hour and a half, four to five times a week, are a great weight-loss strategy. So is building muscle over time. More intense aerobics are fine, as long as they don't tire you out. Some people exercise too much trying to burn calories, and it does not work. All they end up doing is dumping and regaining water and inducing an inflammatory state that plays into the inflammatory problems of leptin and excess body weight. Exercise should always feel good, during and after. A relaxed feeling of improved vitality and energetic function is the answer to how much exercise is right for anyone.

Burning fat during exercise is more likely to occur when you haven't eaten for a while. Thus, an ideal time to exercise is before breakfast or in the afternoon before dinner, assuming you have the energy to exercise at these times without needing to eat. It does not help to exercise when you are already significantly hungry or too tired from not having eaten. If you feel great following exercise you should wait to get a hunger signal before eating, as you are in a prime fat-burning mode.

If you get hungry after exercise you need to eat. If a mealtime is not yet scheduled it is best to move the mealtime up and then eat enough to make it to the next meal. In the future, make sure you eat enough prior to exercise to sustain the demands of the exercise.

Can I Eat Four Meals a Day?

Before trying a four-meal-a-day plan, be sure you are eating properly at your current meals. The most common cause of energy fluctuation during the day is not enough protein at breakfast or at the meal preceding the energy problem. The second most common reason is not enough fat at the last meal. And the third most common cause is too many carbohydrates at the previous meal or earlier that day. For example, fruit juice at breakfast can cause a significant energy drop in the afternoon or out-of-control food cravings after dinner. Pay attention to adequate protein and fat at your meals to ensure you are getting enough of each to help stabilize your energy level. This does not mean excess consumption; it simply means enough to stabilize energy.

In order to produce energy between meals the liver must be in excellent working condition. Some people need to work on liver fitness before they can follow the *Five Rules*. It is permissible to eat four smaller meals a day (300 to 500 calories), spaced four hours apart. This is not ideal, but permissible. As metabolism and energy improve, a person should attempt to go longer between meals, building up "eating fitness."

Problems at Night

Some people feel they must eat something before they go to bed; otherwise, they cannot get to sleep or they feel their sleep will be disturbed by a headache or other symptom of low blood sugar. These issues also relate to the fitness of the liver, as the liver is called on to sustain a constant supply of calories in the blood to maintain blood sugar levels in the normal range. The person needing to eat something before bed has a system that is all wound up and in a stress state.

Just getting the body in a better eating pattern during the day will take stress off the liver, reduce general feelings of emotional stress, and improve nighttime metabolism. When the body feels more relaxed entering sleep, these symptoms will improve. It sometimes takes several months to improve this condition, but it can generally be done by following the *Five Rules* as closely as possible and by getting consistent relaxing exercise, like walking. In the meantime, a person should eat as little as possible before bed and still be able to sleep.

Problems in General

The *Five Rules* are not being used properly if a person experiences troubling symptoms when trying to follow them. The *Five Rules* represent fundamental truth relating to hormones that govern the use of energy in the human body. However, there is no value in inducing some kind of problem or trauma in an attempt to follow them. If troubling symptoms arise from this program, adopt changes more gradually. Work in the direction of being able to follow the *Five Rules*, with the eventual result of feeling great.

Some weight issues are more difficult and require patience and persistence. For example, one common issue for the person who has gained weight is that fat has accumulated in the liver, reducing healthy function. As the individual gradually improves, the excess fat can be metabolized back out of the liver, thus returning liver function to normal. As normal function is achieved it will allow the person to follow the *Five Rules* and feel great.

It can take several months or even longer to correct long-standing metabolic problems. The fact that some of these problems can be corrected at all, simply by eating in harmony with leptin, offers true hope for preventing a relentless spiral into poor health. If you have problems implementing the *Five Rules*, be patient and be consistent. Keep moving in the right direction at a rate your body can handle. You will begin to see improvement in your energy level and symptoms. Even if you feel progress is slow, progress begets progress and builds on itself. Be thankful there is light at the end of the tunnel.

Summary

Some individuals can violate the *Five Rules* and seem to get away with it, but it will catch up with them sooner or later. At minimum, violating these rules is a harder path to follow and creates stress in hormonal systems. The *Five Rules* are a safe and effective way to maintain a healthy eating pattern over the course of a lifetime.

Understanding and implementing the *Five Rules* helps your body form a stable frame of reference for other hormonal and energy patterns in the human body. The *Five Rules* are fundamental for efficiently extracting energy from food—for being able to transform the calorie potential in food to real energy. Energy that can be felt!

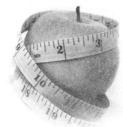

CHAPTER 7

Managing Leptin for Healthy Weight

THE WHOLE PURPOSE OF THE LEPTIN DIET is to create energy and metabolic efficiency in your body. If you are of normal body weight the *Five Rules* will help you extract more energy from less food and maintain your proper weight. If you are overweight, employing the *Five Rules* in conjunction with eating high-quality food and exercising will help to normalize your weight.

When the *Five Rules* are used in an effort to lose weight, they will help you enter a fat-burning mode. This is the metabolic ability to dip into the stores of fat without the body slowing down into a hibernation mode because it thinks it is starving. Diets generally fail because they start out with too much calorie restriction, inducing the starvation response that is almost certain to be followed by weight gain. Another common reason they fail is that they may allow snacking.

Leptin status determines the various modes of metabolic operation in your body. There are five general modes of leptin operation: the balanced-leptin mode, the leptin-resistant mode, the starvation mode, the famine-recovery mode, and the fat-burning mode. When you understand these modes it is much easier for you to maintain healthy metabolic function and enter into and maintain fat-burning mode, as needed.

The Balanced-Leptin Mode

The balanced-leptin mode means leptin is in a condition of equilibrium regarding food intake and energy expenditure; thus, weight is being maintained at a constant. In a truly healthy sense this means your metabolism is running properly, you have a great energy level, and you are of normal body weight.

However, the balanced-leptin mode also can exist in a person of any weight, even a person a hundred pounds overweight. In this situation it simply means that, based on the amount of food eaten, weight is not gained or lost. Leptin, which operates on a subconscious basis, truly believes it is doing a great job. Weight is being maintained at a constant level.

In the balanced-leptin mode, leptin seeks to maintain the *set point* for body weight. In true health, that set point is the ideal body weight. When a person is in a balanced-leptin mode and he or she weighs too much, there is a faulty set point. Consistency in using the *Five Rules* and exercise encourages the set point to drift downward over time. Recalibrating the set point is vital so that weight is not easily gained back following a period of weight loss.

The Leptin-Resistance Mode

The leptin-resistance mode is the most typical mode that dominates in any person who is overweight. It can also occur as a temporary mode, lasting a day or two, in individuals who have just stuffed themselves full, as at a Thanksgiving dinner. It is normal to be able to enjoy a feast from time to time, as part of our social fabric of enjoyment and celebration. A person in good metabolic condition bounces back to normal weight within a day or two. A person stuck in leptin-resistance mode may gain five pounds from eating too much.

The leptin-resistance mode means that excess pounds of fat are generating too much leptin production from fat cells. However, the leptin is not properly entering the brain or registering in the brain, making the body incorrectly think that there is not enough fat in storage. This causes excessive hunger signals and the drive to acquire food, even though the conscious brain realizes such food is not really needed. In this mode there appears to be a lack of willpower or self-discipline to control the urge to eat. Cravings are generally worse at night.

People in this mode are frequently preoccupied with food, constantly thinking about their next meal or what they could be eating now. Obsessions with food may become so intense they ruin a person's life. Even when the consequences of these food problems are adversely influencing an individual's heath or destroying personal relationships, the obsession to acquire food maintains its ranking as one of the subconscious brain's top priorities. This is the leptin nightmare, a place all too familiar to millions of people.

The Starvation Mode

The starvation mode occurs in people who are overweight as well as those who are underweight. The starvation mode is the classic condition of malnutrition, typically accompanied by poor immunity. All anorexic people are stuck in starvation mode as an inflammatory health condition. Individuals can create a starvation mode through excessive exercise, extreme stress, or excessive stimulant intake. The wasting stage of any chronic disease, such as cancer, is always a starvation mode. Fragile health in elderly individuals is typically accompanied by the starvation mode. In essence, the starvation mode is a frail mode, reflected in a feeble energy level, poor immunity, and a trend of bone and muscle loss.

It is quite possible for an overweight person to be stuck in a starvation mode. Such individuals may occasionally crave junk, but it is most common that they have poor appetite and/or experience significant digestive problems when they eat. In general, their metabolism is a casualty of the yo-yo diet war. And even though they signed a peace treaty, they are still getting shot at. The mere thought of going on a diet can cause such a person's metabolism to shut down. The subconscious brain does not trust the person anymore; it never knows when the next hare-brained dieting stunt will take place.

These are the people who already eat a low-calorie diet and still can't lose weight. All their friends are sure they eat junk in private, but these people tend to have almost perfect low-calorie diets. They know that if they begin to eat even the slightest amount of extra food they will begin to gain weight, and once that process is in motion they may gain twenty or thirty pounds before they can bring the weight gain to a stop.

New research is indicating that some of these overweight people have viral infections in their white adipose tissue, which is infecting fat cells, inducing inflammation, and creating a starvation mode due to infectious destruction of the ability of fat cells to make leptin. Yikes, one more nasty angle that may affect a significant number of overweight people who are stuck in a rut.

When overweight people go on a diet, they typically enter into the starvation mode within a few weeks. Thus, weight loss grinds to a halt. The longer they keep trying to diet in a starvation mode, the worse they feel. Energy, mood, and oftentimes immunity simply bottom out. They are often twenty or more pounds from a normal weight and are stuck. While the leptin-resistance mode is a false state of perceived starvation, the starvation mode is true starvation.

The Famine-Recovery Mode

The famine-recovery mode is the mode most hated by any person who has just lost weight. The famine-recovery mode is automatically linked to the back side of the starvation mode. As certain as day will follow night; the famine-recovery mode will follow the starvation mode. It is the mode that has enabled the human race to recover from a period of famine or near starvation; thus, it is hard-wired into the core of genetic survival impulses. It is powerful.

The famine-recovery mode remembers the set point that existed prior to when the person entered the starvation mode.

Thus, if a person was normal body weight prior to a period of food deprivation, the famine-recovery mode will command that as soon as more food is eaten, a greater than normal portion of it will go back to restoring the percentage of body fat that existed prior to the weight loss. Once the brain is satisfied that body fat has been restored, then leptin switches back to the balanced-leptin mode.

In an overweight person, there was a faulty set point prior to the diet that induced the starvation mode. Once the dieting period is over and the person starts to eat more food, even a normal amount of food, the famine-recovery mode clicks on and stays on until the former set point is reached. Unfortunately, the subconscious brain is now even more confused about the set point and very concerned about survival, trusts the person even less. Thus, it may add an extra then to fifteen pounds to the set point as an insurance policy against any future attempts at starvation. Only then does the famine-recovery mode stop, allowing some other leptin mode to take over.

Many people spend their life alternating among the leptin-resistance mode, the starvation mode, and the famine-recovery mode. Their only glimpse of the balanced-leptin mode is at an undesirably high weight. Thus, motivated to take another crack at weight loss, they dive back into the starvation mode and start the cycle all over again.

There is no shortcut to understanding how leptin functions in your personal situation, which may vary under different levels of food intake and stress. There is no single diet that can be handed out to everyone, the list of magical recipes. Fundamental truth regarding diet is rooted in the function of leptin and the quality of food.

The Fat-burning Mode

The fat-burning mode enables a person to maximize the function of leptin so that metabolism can maintain a high level of function while converting excess stored fat into energy. The difference between weight loss that occurs in a starvation mode and weight loss that occurs in a fat-burning mode is that in the proper fat-burning mode the subconscious brain never thinks it is starving.

The *Five Rules* of the Leptin Diet enable leptin and its hormonal management team to smoothly regulate energetic function within the body. Improved efficiency takes significant friction out of the metabolic system, enabling the body to have less inflammation and a faster running, healthy metabolism.

The quality of food is also important. Real quality food, free of toxic hormone disrupters and packing more nutrition per calorie is what the body prefers to see coming in. Poor-quality food is lower in nutritional value and drains energy by inducing digestive challenges.

The combination of the *Five Rules*, high-quality real food, and moderate exercise are the best way to get into fat-burning mode. Fat-burning mode is signified by an excellent energy level in the morning and in the afternoon, cravings that have gone away, a clear head, good sex drive, and weight loss that is gradually occurring.

Some individuals will dump five to ten pounds of water weight while in the first few weeks of fat-burning mode. Consistently maintaining fat-burning mode usually results in two to four pounds of weight loss per month. Faster weight-loss than that, especially if a person feels weak, tired, loses sex drive, or experiences muscle weakness, signals that he or she is actually in starvation mode. Eat enough to stay in an energized fat-burning mode.

Stay on Track

Following the *Five Rules* and accessing fat-burning mode creates a wonderful feeling of energy and well-being. However, when individuals have been in fat-burning mode for a few days and feel great, it does not mean their underlying issues with leptin resistance are solved. They will need to get to an ideal body weight, at which point metabolism will switch to the normal-leptin mode. A person needs to be in normal-leptin mode for a good six months before the new set point is truly in place.

There may be numerous temptations that divert an individual from fat-burning mode. Such temptations cause one to violate one or more of the *Five Rules*. Beware: Fat cells lurk in the wings, ready to refill themselves at a moment's notice. Famine-recovery mode is there waiting to pounce; don't succumb.

Diversions from fat-burning mode typically cost people two to five days of progress. During that time, they will have to wrestle with the additional urges of leptin resistance, previous compulsive-eating urges, and fatigue that did not exist when they were in fat-burning mode.

Summary

People must understand the various modes of leptin in order to know what their metabolism is doing at any given point in time. The ability to lose weight and keep it off is directly related to a personal ability to perceive and correct small changes in metabolism that are heading in the wrong direction. This skill far exceeds basic information about eating less and exercising more. Violations of the *Five Rules* invariably cause problems, sooner or later. You can be in control.

Individuals' rate of progress on the Leptin Diet is governed by their general health as well as their history with weight. I must emphasize, having helped thousands of people, many of whom classified themselves as hopeless weight-loss failures, that the *Five Rules* of the Leptin Diet, high-quality real food, and moderate consistent exercise form the core foundation for everyone and will eventually unravel difficult weight-loss problems. There is no quick fix or magic pill for healthy weight loss.

When you can truthfully answer the question: "Am I happy eating this way the rest of my life?" and you are mainly in balanced-leptin mode at a proper body weight, then you have found a diet that truly works for you. Never take for granted the gift of health.

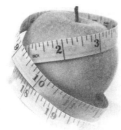

CHAPTER 8

The New Hunter-Gatherer

OUR GOVERNMENT FAILS MISERABLY when it comes to ensuring a high-quality food supply. It now requires considerable skill simply to go shopping. This has led me to coin a new term, the *New Hunter-Gatherer,* reflecting the problems of twenty-first-century food acquisition.

The New Hunter-Gatherer must navigate through the damaged, poisoned, processed, and contaminated food items in order to find a healthful serving of food. It was a far simpler time when what you had to do was shoot something, catch fish in a clean lake or ocean, pick fruit or nuts from a tree, or grow some type of crop.

The majority of our food supply is now produced by large agribusiness. Crops produced by this fast-food farming industry rely on sterilization of insects and weeds through significant applications of chemicals, rather than focusing on the health of the land or the biodiversity of crops. The introduction of genetically modified foods (GMO) tampers with the essence of life in an experiment with an unknown outcome and no real way to undue the damage. The FDA purposely does not require labeling of GMO food, since no one who understands the issue would ever purchase it. This makes it all the more difficult to locate healthful food.

In the fast-food livestock industry, animals live under inhumane conditions and require constant antibiotics to keep their diseases under control. They are fed synthetic growth hormone to rapidly increase their size. Unhealthy animals hold fluid due to inflammation, making them weigh more than healthier animals. Many livestock animals never get exercise, ensuring they will be fatter (profit is by weight). The food produced in this manner apparently needs radiation to kill all the germs resulting from the filthy growing and slaughtering conditions. And now the FDA plans to add bacteria-killing viruses into the food supply to offset contamination risk inherent in poor-quality food production.

Large food-processing companies make significant profits placing crops into boxes while farmers lose money on the same crops. The entire food business is controlled by profits of elite multinational companies—a total racket and monopoly if there ever was one.

We are expected to trust our federal government to determine how much pesticide residue, fungal toxin, antibiotic residue, and pollution in the food supply is safe to consume over the course of a lifetime. Yet we are informed that scientists at the Environmental Protection Agency (EPA) and FDA are routinely overruled by administrators who foster private-sector profits at the expense of public safety. These problems have existed since the birth of the FDA one hundred years ago, an agency that supports monopolistic profiteering and allows numerous chemical adulterations of the food supply. Those wanting to understand the details of this travesty can read my book *Fight for Your Health: Exposing the FDA's Betrayal of America*, as well my numerous articles posted on www.TruthInWellness.com

Pyramid Power

The old and recently retired food pyramid, backed by government agencies, public-health officials, and dieticians was guaranteed to make you fat and unhealthy. My favorite phrase for many years was, "if you eat like a pyramid you will look like one." This old pyramid was a testament to the lobbying skills of vested-interest powers, with lip-service input from dietary experts.

From the point of view of avoiding gaining weight in an out-of-control slide headed for diabetes like a runaway freight train, the new pyramid is better than the old. In a positive direction, the guidelines that accompany the new pyramid tell consumers to avoid trans-fat and refined sugar intake, good steps in the right direction but hardly revolutionary. Anyone taking Nutrition 101 knew these facts fifteen years ago. Why did it take the government so long to acknowledge them?

Politics and Food

The government food pyramid is always an interesting commentary on the politics of our time. The dairy industry has gained new lobbying power, relative to the grain industry. The dairy lobby did quite well in this round of the pyramid power struggle.

We are now supposed to have three glasses of low-fat milk a day. I have nothing against quality milk, but it's not for everyone. People with digestive problems can't process milk well; it simply makes their digestive problems worse. Many Americans don't have the family heritage that supports this much milk consumption. There is also the issue of milk quality. Cows stimulated to produce milk with synthetic bovine growth hormone require constant antibiotics to control their poor health. Typically, such animals are not allowed to freely graze on grass, instead eating moldy corn. If you like milk, buy organic milk from well-treated cows. Keep in mind not all "organic" milk is produced in a quality manner. Consumers need to inquire and be informed about the specific production methods of companies whose food they regularly purchase.

Carbohydrate bashing has taken its toll on the grain industry, although they were thrown a dog bone while being scolded for creating disease. The government still says it is okay to get half your grains from their disease-producing refined carbohydrates. This was a compromise on health, enabling junk-food producers to stay in business poisoning Americans with poor-quality food.

It was very difficult for the vested interests to gain an upper hand among themselves on the subject of protein. Consumers are simply supposed to choose from the various proteins while paying attention to the amount of fat. Actually, most overweight people have no trouble paying attention to the fat. They already know it tastes great and they will be sure to find it on their favorite fast-food menu or pick up the phone and order a pizza. Consumers really don't need the pyramid to guide them.

Meat took a little beating, still having to shrug off the bad reputation it has for being the true evil—saturated fat. Of course, there was no mention that grass-fed beef actually has a very healthful fatty-acid profile conducive to good brain function and metabolism.

The pyramid no longer concerns itself with the number of serving per day. General directions were no longer needed. After the last pyramid got the entire country craving and eating food all day long, the new pyramid simply assumes that people will now eat whenever they want. For those who really need personalized help with this subject, the online pyramid does have a special section you can dive into to get servings per day that are just right for you. If you don't have access to the internet then you'll never have to be burdened trying to figure the pyramid out, since there is no other way for you to learn about it.

The truth is, the government food pyramid has very little to do with your health. It is a policy tool that food-industry segments argue over to determine which companies in the industry will sell the most food to government-run programs such as school lunches—handouts worth billions of dollars. Lip service is given to your health so you think it might have something to do with you. If you don't know the difference between a fat, a carbohydrate, a protein, and water, it may be of some educational value to help clarify these important topics. If you are truly trying to find out what are the best foods to eat or how much of a certain kind of food to consume, you will simply be out of luck.

Choosing Real Food

Food choices are important. You don't need a detailed list. It is not that difficult. You do need a general understanding of the quality of food, the number of calories in various serving sizes, the different types of calories, and how to eat various types of food to sustain your energy.

Think about your entire week. You need variety. You want different kinds of food and you need to eat fruits and vegetables in a wide range of colors. Don't eat the same thing all the time.

Think *flavor*, learn how you can make food taste better. Freshly picked organic produce tastes far better than chemically-tainted and artificially-ripened food. Fresh herbs and spices can bring more taste pleasure to meals, thus reducing the desire to get taste pleasure from servings of fat and sugar. Many condiments contain significant health-promoting properties in and of themselves. Great choices for flavor enhancement include garlic, onions, scallions, cinnamon, ginger, turmeric, basil, cilantro, parsley, oregano, and cloves. Salt is fine in moderation, as long as it does not provoke fluid retention. Avoid MSG and aspartame.

MSG is a neurotoxin. It damages the structure in the brain that is supposed to be registering the leptin signal, which gives a person a normal *full* signal from the proper amount of food. Damaging this brain structure makes the person behave like the mouse that makes no leptin and thus has no normal appetite regulation. There is a reason why there are over fifty studies on the MSG-obese rat in the scientific literature. When scientists need to study a fat rat that is not yet diabetic, they feed it MSG until the rat's brain is so damaged that it eats itself into obesity. When will humans catch on? Considering our huge obesity epidemic, avoiding MSG is essential. The substance should be banned along with aspartame.

Traditional Foods Are the Foundation of Your Eating Plan

Eat foods prepared in the traditional manner of your heritage.

Understand what kind of diet your recent ancestors ate when they were at their healthiest. These foods, prepared in their traditional ways, should form the foundation of your food plan. If you are of European descent, why would you concoct a diet grounded in soy products? If you are of Asian descent, why would you consume dairy products on a routine basis and why would you eat soy that was not prepared as your ancestors prepared the food?

The Power of the Legume

It is a good idea to include legumes as part of your diet. All long-lived healthy cultures have legumes in their diet. In fact, legumes are the only common denominator in all long-lived healthy cultures from around the world. In addition to health-promoting co-factors found in legumes, they help to satisfy the protein requirements of your diet.

While legumes are generally healthy, soybeans may not be. Years ago, during the production of soy oil for a variety of uses, soy protein was thrown away and considered useless. Then the soy industry got the idea to try to sell it at a low price to low-income people. The food tasted so bad that these people would not eat it. Then the industry got the bright idea to sell it as a health food, taking scientific data about soy based on the traditional preparation of the food for a particular ethnic heritage. They superimposed this data onto white middle- and upper-middle-class women of mainly European decent. This sales strategy worked. These women were willing to eat ill-tasting unnaturally prepared soy protein because they were tricked into believing it would reduce their risk of cancer or heart disease.

The truth is that soy protein may induce digestive damage, interfere with thyroid function, and confuse sex-hormone signaling systems. And there is as much data stating that it causes breast cancer as reduces breast cancer. Ninety percent of the soy grown in the U.S. is now genetically modified food. We do not know what the GMO phytoestrogens contained in soy will do when they interact with human breast tissue. Would you like to be part of the experiment? If so, eat soy.

The most common legumes of Mediterranean people are lentils, chickpeas, and white beans. Scandinavians eat more brown beans and peas. Japanese enjoy soy in the form of tofu, natto, and miso. Research now shows that in elderly individuals, for every 80 calories of legumes they have in their daily diet, they reduce their risk of premature death by seven to eight percent. There is no other single component in the Mediterranean diet for which such a claim can be made. There is life force in the legume.

Peanuts are not a nut, they are a legume. The peanut plant comes from South America and is a food product uniquely American. It is potentially a nutritious food. However, peanut butter should show the amount of aflatoxin (a type of mycotoxin) parts per million on the label, as well as the date on which the peanuts were harvested. These omissions prevent the consumer from judging the true quality of this food. Until the labeling of aflatoxin is required, use with caution. Buy peanut butter without added sugar and undiluted with vegetable oils.

Peanuts were not part of the legume study mentioned above. For the purpose of longevity they should not be relied on as the only source of legumes.

Hunting for Red Meat

The New Hunter-Gatherer must learn that all red meat is not the same. Steers raised on grass are eating their traditional diet, and the fat in their meat is quite different from the corn-fed (oftentimes GMO corn) fast-food variety. Steers have special stomachs that convert grass into useful proteins and can modify fats contained naturally in the grass. One thing grass-eaters do is make CLA (conjugated linolenic acid), an important nutrient that supports healthy metabolism. Grass-eaters also concentrate omega-3 oils in their fat, especially the important DHA which is friendly to the heart and vital for brain function. CLA and DHA are missing from the fast-food animals, making them highly inferior in nutritional value.

It takes four to five years for a grass-fed steer to weigh enough to go to market. On the other hand, it takes sixteen months or so to swell a steer to the desirable weight when pumped full of growth hormone and fed junk food. This "cost effective" way of putting meat on the supermarket shelves is a significant compromise in food quality, a difference you can readily taste.

Get a Consistent Dose of Isoprenoids

Whole grains, fruits, and vegetables, contain nutrients known as isoprenoids. Isoprenoids contribute to a plant's flavor and fragrance, regulate germination and growth, and protect the plant from insects and fungus. The flavonoids in deep-colored pigments in fruits, and the carotenes in vegetables, are examples of isoprenoids. Inside cells they perform a rather interesting function, they can deactivate oncogenes (common mutant genes in human cancers), thus reducing the risk for cancer. There is a reason cultures with diets containing fresh fruit, vegetables, and whole grains have lower cancer rates. If you don't eat these foods then you will run low on isoprenoids. This increases the likelihood that mutant cells which cause cancer can get out of control. Ideally these foods should be organic, since organophosphate pesticides are toxic to living cells and work in the exact opposite direction of the health benefits of these otherwise nutritious foods.

Most vegetables qualify as an unlimited food. Eat a variety of colors. Juicing vegetables is okay as long as you get enough other fiber in your diet. However, vegetable juice that contains mostly carrots has too much sugar.

Corn, squash, carrots, and potatoes are higher in sugar content and need to be considered as part of the carbohydrate total of any meal. It is a shame that French fries, potato chips, and corn chips are the mainstay vegetables of the American junk-food diet. Eat these foods in their real forms as part of a real meal. Minimize or avoid them in their junk-food forms.

Carbohydrates from grains should be eaten in as wholesome a form as possible. Highly refined grains are stripped of important nutritional substances that give grains their health value.

The best isoprenoid-containing fruits are signified by their deep color. Excellent choices are blueberries, blackberries, cherries, raspberries, cranberries, pomegranate, and red wine. The colorful pigments of all fruits contain health-promoting nutrients.

Skewed Taste Buds Are a Major Part of the Problem

The taste of simple sugar is a major source of pleasure-based addiction. The tongue has leptin receptors on it that are tuned to sweet taste. When leptin is out of balance, the desire for sweet-tasting foods can be overwhelming. This includes cravings for junk sweets and chocolate, or it may involve cravings for complex carbohydrates such as bread products (especially if they have some kind of sugar on top). Junk-food processors frequently add hidden sugars to their products, which are covered up by other flavors. However, these hidden sugars communicate to the tongue and subconscious brain, confusing leptin and driving the compulsion to eat more food than is needed. The only way to get rid of these excess sweet cravings is to rebalance the leptin receptors on the tongue. When this happens, the desire for the taste of sweets is toned down and the cravings disappear.

Individual perception of sweetness varies considerably from person to person. An adequate level of sweet-taste satisfaction should come from one-two servings of fruit a day, a moderate amount of complex carbohydrates, and an occasional treat for dessert that contains some form of sugar (in a moderate portion). Individuals trying to lose weight are better off skipping all desserts, as their taste buds need to go through addiction withdrawal and get reset to something more normal.

The American Dietetic Association (ADA) thinks you should be able to use any kind of non-calorie sweetener in any amount, at any time of day, so that you can increase the pleasure in your food without increasing the calories. I don't agree. It is best if you avoid all no-calorie sweeteners, because they communicate to the leptin receptors on taste buds and numb them out. This skews taste so that a true *full* signal at future meals is now distorted, thus more calories are eaten. It should be pointed out that the ADA receives large amounts of funding from fast-food agribusiness; as a result, they do not explain true food quality to the American public.

Eat appropriate amounts of real food with moderate sugar calories at mealtimes. Most sugar in the diet should come from fresh fruit and complex whole-grain carbohydrates. Moderation, not deprivation, is the key. If you feel deprived of the taste of sweets from these guidelines, realize you are a sweet addict and have succumbed to the marketing ploys of the vested-interest trash-food monopoly. You have become a pawn in their game of profits at the expense of your health. They are controlling your brain.

After a few months of following the *Five Rules,* you have the chance to recover from this addiction and become normal again. In the meantime, find something else to do besides eating sweets or using sugar alternatives. The problem is your abnormal sense of taste. If you continue to ingest sweet-tasting food in inappropriate amounts or between meals, leptin function will not return to normal.

Do You Consume High-Fructose Diabetic Syrup?

High-fructose corn syrup, in addition to being genetically modified, is devastating to metabolism. The standard diet for making a rat diabetic is to feed it high-fructose corn syrup and excess saturated fat (with no essential fatty acids). Recently, scientists wondered which of these two ingredients was really inducing the diabetes, so they tested them separately. Not surprisingly, they both caused diabetes. Excessive saturated fat piles up in body organs and clogs them to a halt. High-fructose corn syrup causes such severe insulin resistance that diabetes occurs easily. Humans should pay more attention to rat experiments.

Get fructose in moderation from fresh fruit. Don't eat a level of this substance that we have no evolutionary or traditional dietary ability to process. At the levels consumed by sweet-addicted soft-drink consumers, high-fructose corn syrup is poison to the human body and should carry a skull-and-crossbones warning on the label. And since artificial sweeteners confuse leptin receptors, this rules out all soft drinks as part of the Leptin Diet.

The Glycemic Index

The glycemic index is designed to show what foods cause a sugar surge into the blood and thus a rapid rise in insulin. This concept is often referenced as a basic dietary truth for guiding food selection. The glycemic index is overrated. According to it, high-fructose corn syrup would be a good choice for consumers.

This index has some value for understanding how you can eat too many carbohydrates. Studies support the fact that formerly real foods which have had their fiber and nutritional value stripped away are a source of disease. Examples include a diet containing large amounts of white rice or refined grains.

The sugar-raising attributes of any carbohydrate will be modified when eaten with other foods containing fat, protein, or fiber. White potatoes are an example of a real food getting a bad rap. When they are combined with adequate fiber-rich vegetables and other calories in a meal, the sugar surge into the blood is modified. If the meal isn't too large, then the potato is not a problem. If you dump butter and sour cream on the potato, that is another story. And you can buy potatoes that are too large, a natural super-sized portion. The Mediterranean diet, high in vegetables, has always included white potatoes without any adverse health consequence.

If there is any lesson from the glycemic index, it is that diets with a lack of fiber are a huge problem. A person needs 25 grams of fiber per day. Fiber is found in whole grains, fruit, nuts, seeds, vegetables, and legumes. Eating a real-food diet provides the fiber you need. You can always supplement fiber to assist in bowel function and proper clearance of waste products from the digestive tract.

Don't Be Afraid of Fat

Almonds, walnuts, and sesame seeds can offer good nutritional support. These foods, higher in fat along with the protein they provide, need to be considered as part of the total calorie intake of a meal.

Eggs take a lot of abuse. Eggs are an excellent food—as long as they are from range-raised chickens which are fed an organic diet. Almost all individuals can eat eggs regularly if they like them and are not allergic to them. Eggs do not raise cholesterol significantly, if at all, and they do not cause heart disease. In reality, eggs are a heart-friendly food. They contain the highest amount of choline of any commonly eaten food. Choline acts like a fat solvent in the blood, helping to keep fat from sticking together and clogging vital organs. Furthermore, choline makes betaine in metabolism, which helps protect against cholesterol forming plaque in the arteries. Betaine helps clear homocysteine, a known risk factor for hardening of the arteries.

Milk also has a bad name. True enough, some people are allergic to milk or have lactose intolerance, or they just do not like milk. Many people have switched to skim milk because they think the saturated fat in milk will clog their arteries and cause heart disease; even the new pyramid tells them to consume skim milk. A 2004 study from the *British Journal of Nutrition* found milk fat intake is inversely correlated with heart disease and the risk for a first heart attack. In this study insulin levels and leptin levels were lower in relationship to the higher percentage of milk fat in the diet. This means 2% milk is just fine, as long as total calories in a meal don't get too high.

The current studies of milk and eggs do not support that saturated fat or cholesterol from real foods, eaten as part of appropriate-sized meals, pose any risk of heart disease. It is only when these foods are eaten with excessively large meals, especially meals containing refined sugar and refined grain, that the combination becomes a serious health problem. The answer is not to remove or limit excellent foods that truly help provide nutritional value and energy; it is to eat them properly and get rid of the junk that our government, for a number of decades, has been suggesting.

Dairy products are fine in moderation or when consistent with a person's family heritage. Organic is best.

Some Beverages between Meals Are Okay

Clean water is the preferred between-meal beverage, if you are thirsty. Coffee or tea may be used in moderation, especially if a little boost is needed to help keep metabolism moving along. It is okay to have these between meals, as long as no sweetener is added and they do not contain calories in the form of milk or chocolate. If you want cream in your coffee, have it with a meal and count the calories. If you want a latte, have it as part of a meal and count the calories. Generally, do not sweeten coffee or tea.

Caffeine is not for everyone, and too much caffeine will stop weight loss and "wind-up" the metabolic system like a cat on a hot tin roof, leading to overwhelming carbohydrate cravings and inflammatory dehydration. Thus, if drinking a caffeinated beverage between meals makes you eat something before the next proper mealtime, it isn't working for you. Two servings a day is plenty. In some cases this can be very helpful in keeping metabolism moving along; in other cases it is completely un-necessary or may cause problems. You do not need to avoid caffeine on the Leptin Diet, but you need to pay attention to how it affects you. Moderation is the key.

Alcohol in Moderation May or May Not Be Okay

Alcohol with dinner is acceptable if a person responds properly to it. The preferred alcohol is red wine, due to its nutritional benefits. One to two glasses is the maximum. Each glass contains about 125 calories. Reduce complex carbohydrates, if needed, in order not to exceed a proper-sized meal. Some people with leptin problems must abstain from alcohol or drink it only on special occasions. Once they have alcohol, it turns on their pleasure-seeking and food-addiction drive. They lose track of any concept of the proper amount of food and consequently eat too much.

Watch Yourself in a Health Food Store

Health food stores and co-ops, while generally carrying more organic foods, also carry a lot of junk food masquerading as health food. Just because it says organic does not mean you can indiscriminately eat that food in any amount. Many packaged or canned organic foods are fortified with natural cane sugar or some other sugar to get sweet-addicted consumers to buy them. Look at the label and look at the amount of sugar in the product. Don't buy products with added sugar. Then, possibly, the organic industry will quit making them.

Selecting healthy food requires constant vigilance on the part of the New Hunter-Gatherer. The goal of any proper and healthful eating plan is the inclusion of a wide variety of real food in amounts adequate to sustain health.

Support Sustainable Farmers

There is a movement underway to restore our food supply to a state of health. It is a battle being waged by small family farms. They are networking together to form a community of food producers who want to produce high-quality food and make a decent living doing so. It is a battle to maintain financial dignity, a rural way of life, and provide something of true health value to the American people. It is part of our culture. It is a battle of David versus Goliath, and they need our help. Helping is easy—buy their food.

Get to know your local farmers who support the cause of raising and growing food in harmony with nature. It is a lot easier to trust people when you can talk to them. Many cities offer wonderful farmer's markets or other opportunities to get involved, such as delivery of seasonal fresh food to locations in your community. Find out how you can get better-quality food for yourself, and find out what you can do to support farmers. Your personal efforts make a huge difference.

Large food distributors set up contracts with grocery stores and give them better prices for their low-quality meats and many other foods. As part of the deal, these grocers sign agreements that they won't sell locally produced foods in their stores. This is an anti-competition scam that is helping multinational agribusiness destroy our rural communities. The New Hunter-Gatherer has a social responsibility to help change this situation through purchasing decisions. If we don't do this, high-quality food may soon disappear entirely from our food supply.

The guardians of the quality of our food supply are not the federal government, the FDA, the EPA, or multinational agribusinesses. This is like having the fox in charge of the chicken coup. The true guardians are the sustainable family farmers; they are the heroes. And they are hanging on by a thread.

Summary

Making good food choices is truly important. If you make good choices most of the time, then you'll have a little leeway to occasionally diverge. If you make poor choices too often, sooner or later you will drastically impair your health.

The foundation of your diet should be a wide variety of fresh, high-quality foods. Eat in harmony with your family heritage. Learn to understand the number of calories in the foods you typically eat so that you are truly cognizant of meal size. Don't become obsessed with calorie counting and don't be calorie ignorant.

Take the time to relax and enjoy your meals, especially a family gathering for dinner. A person whose metabolism is working well can participate in the occasional feast or celebration. Food is part of culture.

Food is vital for survival. By combining the *Five Rules* with high-quality food, you can maintain a healthy relationship with food and establish the foundation for your right to be healthy. That choice is mostly yours.

The science of leptin is about extracting energy from food. It is far easier to extract energy from quality food. Inherent in low-quality food is the "poison load" that comes along with it, directly interfering with metabolism by inducing inflammation and interfering with hormonal function. The New Hunter-Gatherer must learn to find quality food. It is not an easy task.

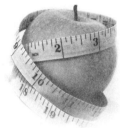

CHAPTER 9

Were You Born to Be Fat?

LEPTIN PLAYS A CRUCIAL ROLE DURING PREGNANCY, in the first few weeks of life, and during childhood. It is involved in numerous activities in addition to appetite and energy regulation and is the key hormone needed for successful reproduction. A common theme for leptin is its pivotal duty of ensuring survival of the human race.

For example, it is well documented that leptin resistance interferes with normal ovulation and can cause infertility. This is especially true if a young woman struggles with obesity and leptin issues during developmental years. Teenage girls who are overweight disturb leptin function as it relates to their female system, an issue with lifelong consequences. Reproductive function is significantly disturbed if obesity starts early, compared to later life onset of leptin problems.

Anorexia is a low-leptin starvation state. The adverse consequences of this eating disorder on reproductive health and fertility are well documented. Women who eat so little or exercise so much that their menstrual cycles are disturbed are also altering leptin function as it relates to their reproductive system. Somewhere between too much food and too little food is the right amount of food to maintain a properly nourished body and healthy reproductive potential. The more a young woman learns the wrong lessons during developmental years, the greater the chances for reproductive problems later in life.

Leptin during Pregnancy

Leptin is the primary hormone that permits healthy pregnancy. During pregnancy leptin levels rise. This promotes the storage of fat so there will be adequate energy reserves to feed the newborn baby. Leptin is also the hormone that enables the placenta to grow. Leptin has a significant impact on the development of healthy nerve and brain function.

Due to the natural rise in leptin levels, pregnancy is a major test of leptin fitness in the mother's metabolic system. This tends to make any already existing leptin-resistance problem worse, in susceptible women it may trigger significant leptin-resistance problems for the first time. Leptin-related problems during pregnancy portend leptin weight issues for the mother following pregnancy.

Many serious problems that occur during pregnancy are caused by leptin-related issues. These include toxemia, high blood pressure, gestational diabetes, hypothyroidism, miscarriage, and premature delivery. The risk for such problems is much higher in a mother who had leptin problems prior to pregnancy, reflected in her struggles with body weight and/or poor thyroid function.

Maternal leptin resistance imposes major stress on the placenta and fetus, potentially altering normal nervous system development. Core development of appetite nerve circuitry may be disturbed, setting the stage for later-life leptin resistance and weight gain in the child. One undesirable result is that leptin problems impose a malnourished impression, a false state of perceived starvation, on the developing nervous system of the fetus. This can result in the failure of the fetus to develop organs to their fullest genetic potential. A common adverse side effect is that kidneys do not develop into their proper size. Later in life, the kidneys will be a weak spot in metabolism for such people, predisposing them to develop high blood pressure and consequent cardiovascular disease.

Individuals with inherently weak leptin "brain wiring" are more susceptible to developing leptin resistance and obesity when challenged by some form of stress to the leptin system. Examples of this stress include the onset of puberty, pregnancy, poor eating habits, or periods of high emotional stress. If weight problems haven't shown up sooner, they will usually become evident in men by age forty and in women at menopause. As hormonal systems age, numerous hormones tend to become resistant or numb, at which point the leptin weakness may become manifest. The consequent weight gain is often very difficult to manage.

We as a society need to place much greater emphasis on the health of women entering childbearing years and during pregnancy. The onset of obesity or eating disorders in teenagers is an ominous black cloud for future generations. Mothers who fail to recover their proper body weight and health vitality before becoming pregnant again are increasing the risk for leptin-driven pregnancy complications, accelerated deterioration of health following pregnancy, and diminished quality of health in their child.

The First Two Weeks of Life

During pregnancy, leptin's role is to sustain pregnancy and aid neurological development. Leptin is not used by the fetus to regulate appetite. The fetus has no full signals and no hunger signals. Connected to mom's food supply by an umbilical cord, the fetus receives a constant influx of nutrition. Upon birth, everything changes.

Nourishment in the first two weeks of life is critical to health over the course of a lifetime. Entering the world, the baby has just been disconnected from his or her food supply and plummeted into a much colder environment. This is a time when leptin and thyroid hormone must work properly to ensure immediate survival as well as establish the first appetite signals to acquire food, signals that will influence an entire lifetime.

The newborn baby requires a dose of leptin to help establish and set up appetite regulation. This critical "first serving" ideally occurs within the first six hours of life. It is provided in the first milk colostrum of the mother. The first job of leptin is to go to the hypothalamus gland of the brain and set up the appetite-control system. This region of the brain is somewhat like a blank chalkboard, as far as appetite is concerned. Yes, healthy leptin function of the mother during pregnancy facilitated the formation of basic brain circuitry; however, now it is time for the infant to establish the first true appetite signals. Leptin writes the first message on the chalkboard, establishing the core hardwiring of the appetite signaling system that will last throughout life.

If a baby does not get first milk colostrum, this important step in brain development does not occur properly. Because most other signals in brain chemistry involve acquiring food, such a child will generally have an inappropriate appetite signaling system and be predisposed to eating too much. In some cases, significant problems won't become evident until later in life, usually triggered by some type of major stress or change in life.

Also in the first milk colostrum is the biologically active thyroid hormone T3. This is needed to help the newborn baby sustain the dramatic growth required in the first two weeks, the adjustment to lower temperatures, and the major development of brain circuitry that must occur in this critical time period.

Other stress factors can interfere with the proper wiring of appetite signals. Premature birth is especially difficult. Overfeeding a low-birth-weight baby can program leptin resistance into the developing brain and result in later-life obesity.

The toxins of an infection or elevated bilirubin (jaundice) are very stressful to developing appetite signals in the subconscious brain. These irritants can literally erase the leptin message from the chalkboard and set the baby up for later problems.

The first two weeks are a critical time that determines immediate survival of the child. The appetite signals formed during this time, along with the gestational nutritional status, are factors that have a major influence on later-life health.

The Developmental Years

Young children's brains have a high level of plasticity. This means that learned behaviors and thought processes are not simply like a computer "software" programs, but are more like hardware. Various lessons of life are imbedded as deeply learned responses.

Children who grow up in malnourished environments may learn to adapt by having a thrifty metabolism, learning to get by on less. However, the scarcity of food and the lack of normal pleasure from adequate food intake tend to be associated with deep-rooted feelings of deprivation. Later in life, these early lessons may become huge problems. Cravings for food and ingestion of excess food overwhelm the thrifty brain circuitry that enabled survival during childhood, leading to obesity in adulthood.

Any childhood stressors that are a threat to survival may disturb the formation of healthy leptin brain circuitry. This is due to leptin's role in deploying energy to manage the stress response. An unhappy or unstable childhood may easily induce stress eating later in life, as a form of pleasure to offset deep-rooted pain. Many adults eat in response to stress, especially if they had a painful childhood; others may eat too often even when they aren't stressed. While they may describe their reason for constant nibbling as boredom, something to do, or a bad habit, further probing typically leads them to describe significant aspects of their childhood as chaotic, unstable, or painful.

Any child who overeats is directly programming leptin resistance into developing brain circuitry. The failure to teach children proper eating rhythms while the nervous system is developing increases the risk for obesity as well as suboptimal brain function. Children with leptin problems automatically develop functional thyroid impairment, since thyroid hormone takes its marching orders from leptin. Impaired function of leptin and thyroid hormones are a considerable disadvantage for the development of intelligence.

Chemical Toxicity

There are a variety of chemical poisons that damage leptin and thyroid function. While many chemicals are known to cause birth defects or cancer, the amount of these poisons required to disrupt metabolism is far lower. There is no question that the chemical contamination of our environment is a major contributing factor to the obesity epidemic.

Sometimes examples are dramatic, as in the case of Felipe Franco, born without arms or legs. Throughout her pregnancy his mother picked pesticide-covered grapes in the fields near her home in Bakersfield, California. The risk of farming and working in the fields with these poisons is associated with increased rates of breast cancer, suicide, infertility, and birth defects. Government investigations into the obvious find no conclusive proof of any harm. Such denial of a problem is a cost-saving benefit handed down to the fast-food farming industry at the expense of human health.

Any pregnant mother eating food that contains residues of these chemicals is putting the health of her child at risk. Organophosphate pesticides are fat-soluble toxins that readily cross the placenta and may adversely affect the developing nervous system of the fetus. These chemicals were invented by the Germans to use as chemical gasses in World War I, and were popularized by the Rockefeller Cartel for use on food following World War II. Today, they are intended to kill pests by destroying their nervous systems. Their safety in humans has been a subject of debate for decades. Due to the vested interests in agribusiness, the EPA cannot get these chemicals out of our food supply. Pregnant women should eat all organic food and avoid contact with any chemical cleaners or chemical pesticides during pregnancy.

PCBs (polychlorinated biphenyls) are a toxin of industrial pollution that contaminates our food supply to this day. It is rapidly absorbed into white adipose tissue and will saturate breast tissue. Not only does this increase the risk for breast cancer in women with a particular genetic susceptibility, these poisons will readily enter the milk supply of the mother. While eating fish from highly contaminated areas poses the greatest risk, PCBs now permeate our land and water. Because they are readily absorbed into fat they disrupt the normal function of leptin in white adipose tissue. Fat-sampling studies have proven that almost all Americans have PCBs in their white adipose tissue. Furthermore, losing weight will release PCBs back into the circulation as fat breaks down, inducing a chemical toxicity. PCBs can induce significant free radical damage. In some cases, the body will not break down "toxic fat," since it is just too poisonous. Such issues complicate weight loss and in some cases halt all progress.

The water supply in many regions of the United States that grow our food is contaminated with perchlorate, a rocket-fuel ignition catalyst used primarily by military contractors. Perchlorate binds to the thyroid gland more tightly than iodine and disrupts metabolism. It is in much of the produce and milk supply of our country. Almost all lettuce contains high amounts of perchlorate. The only way to avoid it is to buy produce grown in regions which do not have a perchlorate-contaminated water supply. The water as well as the food of dairy-producing animals needs to be free of perchlorate. Unfortunately, California, Arizona, Texas, and Florida all have serious perchlorate-contamination issues, polluting the groundwater in large regions of these states. A recent sampling of breast milk taken from mothers at random from around the country showed that all samples were contaminated with perchlorate at levels which could disrupt thyroid function in their infants. Additionally, a newborn or infant drinking perchlorate-contaminated water is at particularly high risk for damage to thyroid function.

These are just a few examples of the adverse effects of environmental poisons on reproduction, as well as on brain development and obesity risk in children. Problems can be passed on for several generations. During the mother's pregnancy, all the eggs of a baby girl that will enable her to be a mother one day are formed while she is still in the womb. Thus, a mother who does everything right during her life and pregnancy to have a healthy child is still partially at the mercy of any problems her own mother had during pregnancy. This is now called the grandma effect. A grandmother who smoked during pregnancy doubles the risk for asthma in her daughter's children.

Exposure to poison over the course of a lifetime is a devastating problem. Many fat-soluble poisons readily accumulate in white adipose tissue, eventually damaging the house in which leptin lives. The consequence is that most overweight people have abnormally high levels of leptin in their blood and have difficulty breaking down fat from various regions of their body because the fat-organ is damaged.

Dangerous Medications

Numerous medications disrupt leptin function, as evidenced by the weight gain that follows their use. Stimulant weight-loss medication also damages leptin function. This can be seen in the weight gain that occurs when such drugs are discontinued. We live in a quick-fix, chemically tainted world that is a major challenge to healthy leptin function.

Relevant to this chapter is the reckless use of brain poisons in our children. Atypical antipsychotic medications, like Zyprexa, are now in widespread off-label use on children, even though they have never been approved for any person under the age of eighteen! These medications are known to induce insulin resistance, weight gain, and diabetes. It is obvious that they seriously disturb leptin function. This problem is sure to have devastating later-life consequences, particularly on the future reproductive function of young women who are gaining weight on these medications.

ADHD medications are stimulant narcotics. They significantly interact with leptin-related brain circuitry, thereby depressing leptin levels while ramping up nerve transmission. Animal studies show that when leptin is depressed by stimulants, brain damage to dopamine nerve structures occurs. Mice that have no leptin are highly susceptible to brain damage from chemicals. Leptin also acts as a significant brain antioxidant.

By abnormally depressing leptin levels in the developing nervous system, nerves are conditioned to improperly respond to appetite signals and are more sensitive to chemical toxicity.

Since children have developing nervous systems, these mistaken lessons are likely to be ingrained in behavior for the rest of their life, setting the stage for later-life obesity. Animal studies indicate that ADHD medication induces lasting brain damage, which is manifested as depression in older animals. Furthermore, if ADHD medications are given to an overweight child, that child already has a lower brain level of leptin due to existing leptin-resistance problems. This means that overweight children will be more likely to suffer adverse neurologic damage from ADHD medications, because they do not have the protection that leptin offers.

Addiction

There is a fine line between healthy pleasure seeking, eating, and addiction. Pleasure in response to doing something is a reward, tied to dopamine function. All such brain circuitry is intimately associated with leptin and appetite. All addictions play off this fundamental drive to survive.

Individuals who develop leptin problems, for whatever reason, are at significantly increased risk for developing addictions to substances (alcohol or drugs) as well as addictive behavioral patterns (sexual compulsion, gambling, shopping). This is because the solution to any "brain pain" or life stress is to get a surge of pleasure as quickly as possible. The pleasure is then associated with the behavior or substance, and it is cross-programmed into the subconscious brain along with the healthy need to acquire food.

Needless to say, food addition itself is a major problem. In some ways it is a chicken-and-egg proposition. For example, leptin problems may set a person up to become an alcoholic, and alcohol abuse always makes leptin problems worse. The widespread use of brain medications in children, medications which produce dopamine surges or alter appetite signals, is setting the stage for later-life problems with addiction.

The apparent need for brain meds in children is no doubt due, at least in part, to poor brain development which has resulted from leptin problems that occurred in the womb and in early childhood. It is quite likely that the medications being used to treat the symptoms of this problem are actually making the underlying problem worse. The price being paid to modulate behavior in the present is trading off on future health. It is no secret that these brain meds commingle with other recreational drugs on the illicit drug market.

Summary

Many weight issues are tied to the personal choice to eat too much and not exercise enough—a self-inflicted epidemic. However, public-health officials who harp on this message are doing little to solve the obesity epidemic. Society needs to learn how to eat to be in harmony with leptin. The food supply needs to be cleaned up. The environment needs to be cleaned up. The widespread use of brain-altering medication in children needs to stop. A new priority needs to be placed on the health of women entering childbearing years, a program that should be a continuation of proper early-life education on the subject.

Those who have caused these problems to our society do not want to foot the bill to correct them, as it will be in the hundreds of billions of dollars. From a societal point of view, either we spend the money now or we spend far more later on the poor health of an aging and leptin-dysfunctional population. The real problem is that a network of companies which profit by creating the current problems are closely allied with a network of companies that will profit by treating all the sick people who are the result. These groups buy political favor at every turn and threaten to sue the government when decisions are made against them; thus, nothing is really done to help the people. Instead, all weight problems are blamed on bad personal choices. This negates the government's responsibility to address this issue from the broader perspective of promoting true health for our citizens.

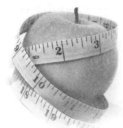

CHAPTER 10

How Fit is Your Fat?

The idea of physically fit muscles is easy to understand. When a person is out of shape, the lack of muscle energy and vitality is obvious. In the same way, any person who gains too much weight is developing unfit fat cells. It is very sobering to realize how bad this problem can become. Unfit fat cells can set in motion a series of energy-crippling metabolic catch-22s that are difficult change. Fatigue is the overriding symptom of unfit fat cells. Diabetes, heart disease, and cancer are the long-term consequences.

Until recently, white adipose tissue had been viewed merely as a storage place for fat. It was thought to have no particular metabolic importance, simply a warehouse for extra calories. The discovery of leptin changed this view. Most researchers now think of white adipose tissue as a metabolic organ, like the liver, heart, and kidneys. This tissue is composed of both fat cells and immune cells. About thirty percent of the cells in white adipose tissue are immune cells.

Scientists have discovered numerous metabolic signals coming from both the fat cells and the immune cells in white adipose tissue. Leptin is the hormone of greatest importance produced by the fat cells. An inflammatory signal called TNFa is the most important signal, for the purpose of this discussion, produced by the immune cells contained in white adipose tissue. As a person gains weight and develops extra pounds of white adipose tissue, there is an increased production of leptin and TNFa simply because there are more pounds of fat on hand.

Extra TNFa coming from extra pounds of fat is like having an argument with someone twenty-four hours a day, seven days a week. It induces major wear and tear, on top of any other wear and tear. All diseases of aging are rooted in excess inflammation. Thus, extra pounds of fat directly contribute to or cause these diseases.

Fat Cells Bulging at Their Seams

The problem of unfit fat cells begins with excess calorie consumption. This causes fat cells to swell in size to accommodate the surplus calories that are not used by the body. Some of this is okay, as fat cells can accommodate varying amounts of fat. There is a fat cell "tone," similar to the idea of muscle tone. It enables the fat cell to swell a bit to accommodate extra fat and shrink down again as fat is used.

Once a line is crossed and there is too much fat in the fat cell, one option is for the fat cells to start making more fat cells in order to store the excess fat coming to them. This of course causes the white adipose tissue to grow, including an increase in inflammation-producing immune cells. Fat cells are fairly adept at dividing and growing, leading to an increase in the amount of white adipose tissue.

Each fat cell also possesses metabolic capability. As leptin levels rise in white adipose tissue, leptin receptors within the fat cell are activated. In a normal-weight and healthy person, this activation tells the fat cell that general nutritional status for the body is acceptable. The activated leptin receptors then release triglycerides stored within fat cells to use for energy.

An unfit fat cell is so crammed full of triglycerides that the leptin receptors are actually clogged by physical pressure, blocking leptin from binding to the leptin receptors inside the cells. The result is that no fat is being released and no weight is being lost.

A simple way to gauge the amount of unfit fat cells is to measure your waistline. The type of fat in the abdominal region is the most closely associated with disease risk, meaning that this type of fat cranks out higher amounts of inflammatory TNFa, which in turn provokes excessive free radical damage. Abdominal fat is a highly accurate predictive indicator of developing fat in other wrong places. These include marbleizing the liver and muscles, congesting the pancreas, or forming plaque in the arteries.

Body tissues containing excess fat look more like a piece of bacon than like a slice of lean beef. Any cell or organ can be clogged with excess fat, which results in impaired function. Organs that are susceptible to excessive free radical damage, such as the liver, are at risk for having the excessive fat "cooked" by free radicals. The liver eventually ends up looking like a charred slice of bacon, otherwise known as cirrhosis of the liver.

The waistline measurement indicating a serious problem is 33 to 35 inches and above for women (28 or less is best) and 37 to 40 inches and above for men (34 or less is best). The taller an individual, the higher the number before significant disease risk starts, generally reflecting a larger body frame. The lower end of this range applies to shorter individuals. A flat tummy is definitely the best for anyone.

Elevated Cholesterol

One main reason for elevated cholesterol in overweight individuals is the unfit fat cell. Bulging fat cells are very unstable, on the verge of rupturing and dying. All cell membranes in the human body are stabilized by fragments of cholesterol, their natural foundation. Unfit fat cells, in a state of panic, send a distress signal to the liver to raise cholesterol production. The liver then sends cholesterol to white adipose tissue in order to stabilize the unfit cells.

Unfortunately, the cholesterol that is made and sent to the fat cells is not able to fix them. Thus, unfit fat cells send a chronic signal to the liver to raise cholesterol. Medications to lower cholesterol do not solve the source of this problem. This problem only goes away when the fat cells shrink in size.

High Blood Pressure

High blood pressure is often caused by unfit fat cells. Adrenaline released from the nerves stimulates white adipose tissue to break down fat. When fat cells become unfit, the body yells at them, trying to get some proper energy out of them. Unfortunately, the yelling is done with excess adrenaline. The unfit fat cells have gone numb to adrenaline, but the circulatory system and kidneys have not.

Excess adrenaline is particularly hard on the kidneys and circulatory system. Adrenaline tends to turn up the force behind circulation, like opening up the faucet so that more water will flow out faster. This is useful for meeting emergency demands in the short term. However, when adrenaline is in the unhealthy pattern of trying to stimulate numb fat cells on a daily basis, it is very hard on the kidneys and creates significant inflammatory tension in the circulation. Eventually, this leads to high blood pressure and hardened, plaque-filled arteries.

There is nothing wrong with salt, in and of itself. Healthy kidneys can easily handle significant or varying amounts of sodium consumption. Those who notice increased swelling or elevated blood pressure when they consume too much salt have a weakened kidney system. This is consistent with out-of-shape fat cells.

Fluid Retention

Fluid retention in overweight individuals is another sign of unfit fat cells. Some types of fluid retention are obvious. Rings become tighter at night. There may be sock lines on the legs from fluid buildup. Fluid buildup requires the heart to exert more pressure tension in order to force circulation of nutrients to sluggish and stagnant areas of the body. This also leads to high blood pressure.

The extra TNFa coming from metabolically unfit white adipose tissue is a significant contributing factor to inflammation.

As part of its natural defense system, the body holds onto excess water to cool off the inflammation, like putting miniature ice packs on cellular sprained ankles. This means that water can be held everywhere, simply for the purpose of cooling off hot and inflamed body tissue.

Fluid-retention problems are typically made worse by excess carbohydrate consumption. The normal way muscles rehydrate and refuel themselves is to transport water and sugar in tandem. When a person eats too many carbohydrates the sugar attracts water; yet the muscles don't need the sugar so it ends up contributing to fluid retention. This is why some people drop five to ten pounds in the first week on a diet low in carbohydrates. Such weight loss is mainly fluid that was being held in a stagnant condition.

The easiest way to judge this problem is to stand on the scale in the morning and again at night. People who weigh two pounds or more at night either ate too many carbohydrates, had too much inflammation that day (stress of one type or another), or have an underlying health problem that is too inflammatory. Regardless of the reason, weight loss will not occur under this condition.

Most individuals who take diuretics for fluid retention or blood pressure have tremendous difficulty losing weight. This is because diuretic medication disturbs electrolyte balance and contributes to the de-energized fat-cell issue. On the other hand, if they don't take the diuretics then fluid will build up easily—a reflection of how out of shape their fat cells actually are. As fat cells get back in shape, the need for diuretics goes away, a true sign of health improvement.

Many individuals only like to weigh themselves following aerobic exercise that involved sweating. This is a time they dump excess water. A key question becomes, Do they gain all the water weight back the next time they eat? Individuals can exhaust themselves trying to lose weight with excess exercise when all they are doing is dumping and regaining water. The real problem is unfit fat cells reflected by a wear-and-tear inflammatory state. Such people would do better with long walks rather than intense exercise.

The Failure to Lose Weight

Another sign of the unfit fat cell is a person's failure to lose weight even when controlling calorie intake and exercising. In a generally healthy person, body weight will start to drop when calories are reduced and exercise is increased. This is especially true if the person is eating in harmony with leptin and following the Five Rules. In many cases, just eating in harmony with leptin will get weight loss back on track, even in people who say nothing works for them.

There are people who struggle to lose weight even though they are following the Five Rules, eating a proper amount of calories, and exercising. Such individuals have a significant case of metabolically unfit fat cells. They may also have key body organs that are clogged with fat, and their brain circuitry relating to leptin may not be in good working condition.

Commonly, inflammation generated in an effort to get through the day will grind weight loss to a halt. This typically feels like one's energy level is declining by the afternoon and it is an effort to push through the day. Emotional stress makes this worse, but the demands of the day in themselves may induce wear and tear that hobbles metabolism.

In this situation it is risky to use stimulants to try to lose weight; these include diet drugs, boosting up thyroid medication, and increasing caffeine ingestion. Such strategies may work minimally in the short term, but they add considerable stress to the kidneys and may aggravate other problems discussed in this chapter.

The best lifestyle adjustment is to lessen physical and emotional demands during the day and to take longer walks. Intense exercise tends to induce too much inflammation, which is already a problem. Longer walks tend to increase endorphins, which reduce inflammation and stimulate the liver to burn fat. Unfortunately, many individuals do not have the luxury to decrease their physical or emotional demands. Until they figure out a solution for their own situation it is unlikely that they will lose weight.

Summary

The problem of unfit fat cells tends to become worse as time goes along. The first sign of the problem is gaining weight that is difficult to lose when calories are reduced and exercise is increased. This weight gain is typically in the abdominal area.

As the problem worsens other problems crop up. One or more of the following is typical: elevated cholesterol, high blood pressure, and/or fluid retention. As the problem really sets in, the demands of the day induce fatigue too easily; this, in turn, plays off these other problems and locks them into place.

Following the Five Rules of the Leptin Diet will often enable a person to get back on track and slowly yet steadily correct these problems and lose weight. If needed, a person may have to figure out a way to reduce the demands of life in order to have the time and energy to benefit from long and relaxing walks.

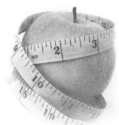

CHAPTER 11

Leptin and Disease

MANAGING LEPTIN PROPERLY OVER THE COURSE OF A LIFETIME provides the best hope for living a disease-free life. White adipose tissue that is in poor physical fitness, along with progressive deterioration of leptin function, inevitably leads to the early onset of the diseases of aging. This includes all forms of cognitive decline, diabetes, cancer, and cardiovascular disease.

Leptin-related problems are now recognized as a primary cause of the number-one killer in America, cardiovascular disease. Heart disease and stroke account for forty percent of all deaths each year. The real problem is that Americans are falling into risk patterns for developing cardiovascular disease at earlier ages. This leads to years of poor health, robbing individuals of the quality of their lives.

It is now widely recognized that ongoing inflammation takes its toll on the physical body and leads to a state of deterioration that is eventually recognized as disease. Any strategy that lowers inflammation will improve health. Many factors are involved. Some factors are mainly under your control, including getting adequate sleep, eating well, getting refreshing exercise, and managing stress. Other factors are more difficult, such as pollution, adulteration of the food supply, and overuse of prescribed medications.

The bottom line for everyone is how well they manage inflammation over the course of a lifetime. Youth proclaims invincibility. Middle age sees the handwriting on the wall. Patterns are deeply rooted, taking hold in the womb and then setting a foundation for the future during childhood. Will the elderly look back over their lives and survey the damage done, or will they enjoy their health and share their wisdom? What type of future are we making possible for our children and grandchildren?

Inflammation Is Necessary

Inflammation is an essential aspect of human function. However, when inflammation becomes excessive, even on a low-grade basis, over an extended period of time, then major problems occur to human health. While many individuals can understand the inflammation of a nagging ache or pain, it is more difficult to understand micro-inflammation occurring at the cellular level or along the lining of arteries. This is mainly felt as fatigue and as a progressive feeling of wear and tear. Muscles tighten up too easily under the influence of low-grade inflammation, leading to stiff shoulders and an overall lack of flexibility. In some ways, chronic low-grade inflammation is a silent problem. Yet the absence of the feeling of vibrant health is a telling sign that difficulties are brewing.

Healthy function involves an ebb and flow of inflammation and anti-inflammation. The inflammatory wear and tear generated by getting through the day is offset by restorative sleep that night. An injury, like a sprained ankle, is always met with inflammation, and then followed by healing. Cells regulate inflammation on their surfaces based on the fatty acids that comprise cell membranes; the higher the omega-3 oils in cell membranes the greater the ability to manage inflammation. Inside cells, inflammation is managed by the antioxidant reserves of a cell. Poor diet dramatically reduces cellular defense systems and tilts them into an ongoing low-grade inflammatory condition, predisposing a person to disease. The human body has a tremendous capacity to withstand abuse, but cellular wear and tear eventually takes its toll.

The Leptin-Disease Link

Inflammation is coordinated by the immune system, which in addition to defending the body against foreign invaders is in charge of repair function. Leptin itself, while considered a hormone, is structured as an immune system messenger (cytokine). Thus, leptin can directly induce inflammation as well as reduce inflammation, depending on what the body needs at any given time. Unfortunately, when problems with leptin occur, leptin directly induces excessive and chronic low-grade inflammation in the circulatory system. Scientists have determined that higher blood levels of leptin induce elevated C-reactive protein (CRP), a condition commonly occurring in obesity and a known risk factor for heart disease.

This is complicated by the fact that an overweight person has excessive numbers of immune cells in the white adipose tissue that are also generating inflammation. The primary inflammatory signals are TNFa and IL 6 (interleukin 6). Some of this inflammation stays localized in the white adipose tissue, leading to damage of this vital organ. However, the accumulation of excess fat, especially fat in the abdominal area, leads to an increase of low-grade inflammation throughout the entire body. This is a significant source of wear and tear, leading to eventual disease. It is now well recognized in the scientific literature that obesity is an inflammatory condition.

A variety of new studies (listed in the appendix) show that leptin problems are a primary risk factor for a first heart attack and first stroke. Numerous studies conclusively demonstrate that leptin problems raise cholesterol, elevate blood pressure, cause blood cells to stick together too easily, and induce kidney damage.

Leptin receptors have now been found on the heart itself. Leptin is involved with the proper energetic function of the heart as well as with blood cells in the circulation. In other words, leptin is intimately involved with multiple aspects of cardiovascular function. Leptin problems are a primary risk factor for the development of cardiovascular disease. The only other factors that may be as bad are chemical toxins in our food, water, and air, or those intentionally ingested (smoking). The combination of chemical toxins and leptin problems is a recipe for disease.

Are Drugs the Answer?

Recently I was interviewed by a reporter from the Wall Street Journal who was doing an article on leptin (The New Thing in Dieting, April 4, 2006, WSJ). She began the conversation by saying, "I've got some bad news for you. I've talked to the scientists who discovered leptin, and they say leptin is not influenced by the diet." I said, "What drug company are they working for?"

Imagine, the hormone that regulates food intake and enables our race to survive starvation not being influenced by diet.

I've got some bad news for these Big Pharma scientists; "None of you will ever make a leptin drug that safely and effectively helps people lose weight."

The thousands of studies done on leptin are mainly intended to figure out how to make drugs to combat obesity. Humans don't have a lack of leptin. What we are lacking is the efficient function of the hormone in our bodies. Most of that problem is induced by diet. Some of the problem is from fetal programming and childhood lessons. The rest of it is induced by toxins.

Big Pharma is spending hundreds of millions of dollars trying to figure out how to modulate leptin or one of its coexisting appetite signals. The problem in designing drugs is clear: these signals are all intimately interwoven with survival. Drugs that influence them have major adverse side effects to human health and metabolism, like taking a sledgehammer to a fly.

Right now, Big Pharma is trying to slip a leptin drug onto the market for the treatment of anorexia, which is an inflammatory low-leptin condition. Their plan is to sneak the drug onto the market for a condition which it might help, and then widely promote its off-label use for weight loss. Sadly, only then will the majority of doctors in America develop even a rudimentary understanding of leptin. Even worse, many unsuspecting consumers will be injured.

Leptin is the master hormone controlling energy for the entire body. It has daily patterns, meal-related timing, and minute-by-minute tone in the circulatory system. It regulates immunity and reproduction. Its complexity of function is mind-boggling. No leptin drug or drug to control the appetite will ever restore normal health.

Your Path to Health

There is no quick fix for leptin problems. You must restore leptin to its rightful position, enabling it to do its job as commander in chief of the hundred trillion cells that comprise your body.

The great majority of people will improve simply by following the Five Rules of the Leptin Diet and eating higher-quality food at their meals. People struggling with metabolism and body weight will need to learn the ins and outs of leptin function and how they apply on an individual basis. This book contains a basic road map. My earlier book Mastering Leptin (which is continuously revised), provides insights into unraveling more difficult problems, such as stubborn weight loss and fibromyalgia.

The good news is that one does not have to be perfect for there to be a significant reduction in disease risk. Once a person gets into a healthy eating pattern, starts losing weight, and is headed consistently in the right direction≠—risk factors for cardiovascular disease significantly decline. This is because the raging fire of inflammatory leptin problems has been temporarily extinguished in the circulatory system. However, until all extra weight is lost, these problems still exist in the white adipose tissue and can flare up anytime a person gets off track.

Managing leptin consistently over the course of a lifetime is like discovering the pot of gold at the end of the rainbow. Your reward is a healthy life and growing older with your health intact.

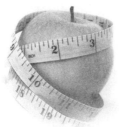

Leptin Science

I HAVE SELECTED KEY STUDIES that explain how leptin functions, the scientific foundation of the *Five Rules* of the Leptin Diet, and the health consequences of not solving this vital health issue. In particular, I focus on cardiovascular disease, explaining how leptin problems are a major factor in the number-one killer in America. I give brief explanations so that you will know what these studies are about. If you would like to look up the details of a particular study, you can find them on PubMed (http://www.ncbi.nlm.nih.gov/entrez/query.fcgi).

In 2002, when I first published *Mastering Leptin*, there were over five thousand leptin studies. As of October 2006, there are over eleven thousand. I was the first author to explain leptin to the general public, as well as how to eat in harmony with leptin in order to lose weight and maintain a healthy weight. I also explained the details of how leptin problems cause many types of cancer. In addition to the references below, there are hundreds more references listed in *Mastering Leptin* that support the work in that book, which is still valid today.

Leptin, originating in fat cells, travels to the brain, where it regulates energetic function for the entire body. In the hypothalamus gland, leptin establishes a set point for weight. It is also acts like a traffic cop, allowing metabolism to run and enforcing how fast it can run. In healthy people, when adequate fat is in storage, metabolism runs faster. These studies explain this basic function.

A) Friedman JM. The function of leptin in nutrition, weight, and physiology. *Nutr Rev.* 2002 Oct;60(10 Pt 2):S1-14; discussion S68-84, 85-7.

B) Meister B. Control of food intake via leptin receptors in the hypothalamus. *Vitam Horm.* 2000;59:265-304.

C) King PJ. The hypothalamus and obesity. *Curr Drug Targets.* 2005 Mar;6(2):225-40.

D) Arch JR. Central regulation of energy balance: inputs, outputs and leptin resistance. *Proc Nutr Soc.* 2005 Feb;64(1):39-46.

E) Havel PJ. Role of adipose tissue in body-weight regulation: mechanisms regulating leptin production and energy balance. *Proc Nutr Soc.* 2000 Aug;59(3):359-71.

F) This study explains that appetite is regulated primarily by leptin, with input from numerous other signals. Bringing these signals into harmony is a key reason why factors such as meal size and meal timing are so important to proper leptin function (not just total calorie intake in a day). Halford JC, Cooper GD, Dovey TM. The pharmacology of human appetite expression. *Curr Drug Targets.* 2004 Apr;5(3):221-40.

The most basic leptin problem is called *leptin resistance*. It means leptin does not enter the brain. One reason for this is that high triglycerides in the blood, from excess eating, are blocking entry to the brain. The body starts to think it is starving. As problems set in, fat cells expand and get clogged, another way leptin is disturbed. Swollen fat cells signal the liver to make extra cholesterol. Improper dieting (starvation) may induce weight loss; however, it is invariably followed by weight gain.

A) Banks WA, Coon AB, Robinson SM, Moinuddin A, Shultz JM, Nakaoke R, Morley JE. Triglycerides induce leptin resistance at the blood-brain barrier. *Diabetes.* 2004 May;53(5):1253-60.

B) Jequier E. Leptin signaling, adiposity, and energy balance. Ann N Y Acad Sci. 2002 Jun;967:379-88.

C) Fan X, Bradbury MW, Berk PD. Leptin and insulin modulate nutrient partitioning and weight loss in ob/ob mice through regulation of long-chain fatty acid uptake by adipocytes. *J Nutr.* 2003 Sep;133(9):2707-15.

D) This study shows increased cholesterol due to larger fat-cell membranes. Shimano H. Sterol regulatory element-binding protein family as global regulators of lipid synthetic genes in energy metabolism. *Vitam Horm.* 2002;65:167-94.

E) The lower leptin goes during weight reduction, the higher the likelihood of a relapse. Celi F, Bini V, Papi F, Contessa G, Santilli E, Falorni A. Leptin serum levels are involved in the relapse after weight excess reduction in obese children and adolescents. *Diabetes Nutr Metab.* 2003 Oct-Dec;16(5-6):306-11.

F) Leptin seeks to maintain the set point and is the typical reason why diets fail following a period of reduced calorie intake, causing weight regain. Tounian P. [Body-weight regulation in children: a key to obesity physiopathology understanding][Article in French]*Arch Pediatr.* 2004 Mar;11(3):240-4.

Leptin problems cause inappropriate pleasure desire for food, paralleling addiction brain chemistry. Such addictions are "memorized" as learned behavior.

A) Food addiction is real. Del Parigi A, Chen K, Salbe AD, Reiman EM, Tataranni PA. Are we addicted to food? *Obes Res.* 2003 Apr;11(4):493-5.

B) Drive to acquire food is based on dopamine. Szczypka MS, Rainey MA, Palmiter RD. Dopamine is required for hyperphagia in Lep(ob/ob) mice. *Nat Genet.* 2000 May;25(1):102-4.

C) Leptin regulates dopamine; high leptin causes excess food cravings. Krugel U, Schraft T, Kittner H, Kiess W, Illes P. Basal and feeding-evoked dopamine release in the rat nucleus accumbens is depressed by leptin. *Eur J Pharmacol.* 2003 Dec 15;482(1-3):185-7.

D) A surge in dopamine gives a pleasure-reward signal. Volkow ND, Li TK. Drug addiction: the neurobiology of behaviour gone awry. *Nat Rev Neurosci.* 2004 Dec;5(12):963-70.

E) The brain alters its physical structure to seek the substance (food). Winder DG, Egli RE, Schramm NL, Matthews RT. Synaptic plasticity in drug reward circuitry. *Curr Mol Med.* 2002 Nov;2(7):667-76.

F) The addictive pattern is memorized. Nestler EJ. Common molecular and cellular substrates of addiction and memory. *Neurobiol Learn Mem.* 2002 Nov;78(3):637-47.

Sugar is the fundamental addiction

A) Leptin is excessively stimulated by the amount of sugar in a meal. Levy JR, Stevens W. Plasma Hyperosmolality Stimulates Leptin Secretion Acutely by a Vasopressin - Adrenal Mechanism. *Am J Physiol Endocrinol Metab.* 2004 Apr 6

B) Leptin receptors on tongue responds to sweet taste, altering behavior. Shigemura N, Ohta R, Kusakabe Y, Miura H, Hino A, Koyano K, Nakashima K, Ninomiya Y. Leptin modulates behavioral responses to sweet substances by influencing peripheral taste structures. *Endocrinology.* 2004 Feb;145(2):839-47. Epub 2003 Oct 30.

C) Sugar or drug rewards enforce addictive conditioning. Di Ciano P, Everitt BJ. Conditioned reinforcing properties of stimuli paired with self-administered cocaine, heroin or sucrose: implications for the persistence of addictive behaviour. *Neuropharmacology.* 2004;47 Suppl 1:202-13.

D) Learned addiction. Wang GJ, Volkow ND, Thanos PK, Fowler JS. Similarity between obesity and drug addiction as assessed by neurofunctional imaging: a concept review. *J Addict Dis.* 2004;23(3):39-53.

E) The American Dietetic Association ignores sweet-related addiction (contributing to obesity). American Dietetic Association. Position of the American Dietetic Association: use of nutritive and nonnutritive sweeteners. *J Am Diet Assoc.* 2004 Feb;104(2):255-75.

Thyroid hormone malfunctions in response to leptin problems

A) Leptin resistance causes "false starvation" that slows thyroid function even though a person is overweight. Huo L, Munzberg H, Nillni EA, Bjorbaek C. Role of signal transducer and activator of transcription 3 in regulation of hypothalamic trh gene expression by leptin. *Endocrinology.* 2004 May;145(5):2516-23. Epub 2004 Feb 5.

B) Inflammation from fat cells can inactivate the conversion of T4 to active T3. Nagaya T, Fujieda M, Otsuka G, Yang JP, Okamoto T, Seo H. A potential role of activated NF-kappa B in the pathogenesis of euthyroid sick syndrome. *J Clin Invest.* 2000 Aug;106(3):393-402.

C) Reduced thyroid function causes cells to store fat and raise cholesterol. Shin DJ, Osborne TF. Thyroid hormone regulation and cholesterol metabolism are connected through Sterol Regulatory Element-Binding Protein-2 (SREBP-2). J Biol Chem. 2003 Sep 5;278(36):34114-8. *Epub 2003* Jun 26.

D) Truly low leptin levels (malnutrition or diet induced), characteristic of the starvation mode, always cause low thyroid, poor reproductive function, and reduced growth hormone. Chan JL, Mantzoros CS. Role of leptin in energy-deprivation states: normal human physiology and clinical implications for hypothalamic amenorrhoea and anorexia nervosa. *Lancet.* 2005 Jul 2-8;366(9479):74-85.

E) It is clear that leptin levels must be high enough to permit activation of sex-hormone and thyroid-hormone function. Bluher S, Mantzoros CS. The role of leptin in regulating neuroendocrine function in humans. *J Nutr.* 2004 Sep;134(9):2469S-2474S.

F) As healthy men enter a too restrictive diet, thyroid-hormone and sex-hormone systems are significantly reduced in function. Chan JL, Heist K, DePaoli AM, Veldhuis JD, Mantzoros CS. The role of falling leptin levels in the neuroendocrine and metabolic adaptation to short-term starvation in healthy men. *J Clin Invest.* 2003 May;111(9):1409-21.

Women have higher leptin than men to allow a higher percentage of body fat to sustain reproduction. Proper leptin function is vital for healthy reproduction and the future health of a child. The health of women of reproductive age has a tremendous bearing on the future health of society.

Obesity and leptin problems cause major issues with reproductive health, including infertility and failed fertility treatment.

Bellver J, Busso C, Pellicer A, Remohi J, Simon C. Obesity and assisted reproductive technology outcomes. *Reprod Biomed Online.* 2006 May;12(5):562-8.

Leptin problems directly interfere with proper ovarian function and reproductive health.

A) Pasquali R, Gambineri A. Metabolic effects of obesity on reproduction. *Reprod Biomed Online.* 2006 May;12(5):542-51.

B) ESHRE Capri Workshop Group. Nutrition and reproduction in women. *Hum Reprod Update.* 2006 May-Jun;12(3):193-207. Epub 2006 Jan 31.

Leptin problems in obese women induce serious health risks during pregnancy.

Ramsay JE, Ferrell WR, Crawford L, Wallace AM, Greer IA, Sattar N. Maternal obesity is associated with dysregulation of metabolic, vascular, and inflammatory pathways. *J Clin Endocrinol Metab.* 2002 Sep;87(9):4231-7.

During preganancy, leptin problems cause pre-eclampsia.

Lu D, Yang X, Wu Y, Wang H, Huang H, Dong M. Serum adiponectin, leptin and soluble leptin receptor in pre-eclampsia. *Int J Gynaecol Obstet.* 2006 Aug 17; [Epub ahead of print]

A mother's leptin problems during pregnancy have a major influence on later-life disease risk in the child.

Stocker CJ, Arch JR, Cawthorne MA. Fetal origins of insulin resistance and obesity. *Proc Nutr Soc.* 2005 May;64(2):143-51.

New insights are unraveling how leptin and fetal programming cause low-birth-weight babies and consequent increased diabetes, obesity, and cardiovascular risk.

Cripps RL, Martin-Gronert MS, Ozanne SE. Fetal and perinatal programming of appetite. *Clin Sci* (Lond). 2005 Jul;109(1):1-11.

Low birth weight babies at higher risk for metabolic and cardiovascular disease.

Luo ZC, Fraser WD, Julien P, Deal CL, Audibert F, Smith GN, Xiong X, Walker M. Tracing the origins of "fetal origins" of adult diseases: Programming by oxidative stress? *Med Hypotheses.* 2005 Sep 26; [Epub ahead of print]

Low birth weight babies are at higher risk for later-life diabetes.

Martin-Gronert MS, Ozanne SE. Programming of appetite and type 2 diabetes. *Early Hum Dev.* 2005 Dec;81(12):981-8. Epub 2005 Oct 27.

It is vital for a newborn baby to get a first serving of leptin from colostrum, to help program proper appetite signals.

Locke R. Preventing obesity: the breast milk-leptin connection. *Acta Paediatr.* 2002;91(9):891-4.

Leptin levels are higher in breast fed children due to the presence of leptin in breast milk, needed for growth and developing proper appetite regulation.

Savino F, Nanni GE, Maccario S, Costamagna M, Oggero R, Silvestro L. Breast-fed infants have higher leptin values than formula-fed infants in the first four months of life. J Pediatr Endocrinol Metab. 2004 Nov;17(11):1527-32.

Leptin signals the start of puberty.

Kelesidis T, Mantzoros CS. The emerging role of leptin in humans. *diatr Endocrinol Rev.* 2006 Mar;3(3):239-48.

Early puberty is triggered by leptin-driven obesity.

Tam CS, de Zegher F, Garnett SP, Baur LA, Cowell CT. Opposing Influences of Prenatal and Postnatal Growth on the Timing of Menarche. *J Clin Endocrinol Metab.* 2006 Aug 22; [Epub ahead of print]

Improvement of menstrual cycle function in school-age children through the prevention of obesity from a public health education program, predicting lower breast cancer.

Chavarro JE, Peterson KE, Sobol AM, Wiecha JL, Gortmaker SL. Effects of a School-based Obesity-prevention Intervention on Menarche (United States). Cancer Causes Control. 2005 Dec;16(10):1245-52.

The genetic mechanism on how leptin resistance and obesity cause breast cancer is now more fully identified.

> Fortuny Mdel C, Diaz BB, Cabrera de Leon A. Leptin, estrogens and cancer. *Mini Rev Med Chem.* 2006 Aug;6(8):897-907.

As weight is gained, white adipose tissue grows in size. Immune cells within the white adipose tissue (about 30% of the cells that comprise white adipose tissue), called *adipokines*, release highly inflammatory signals that cause health problems for the entire body. These leptin-driven inflammatory problems correlate with increased risk of death in the elderly, especially from heart disease. Diet is a key to preventing these problems.

> A) Lee YH, Pratley RE. The evolving role of inflammation in obesity and the metabolic syndrome. Curr Diab Rep. 2005 Feb;5(1):70-5.
>
> B) Trayhurn P, Wood IS. Adipokines: inflammation and the pleiotropic role of white adipose tissue. *Br J Nutr.* 2004 Sep;92(3):347-55.
>
> C) Das UN. Is obesity an inflammatory condition? *Nutrition.* 2001 Nov-Dec;17(11-12):953-66.
>
> D) Trayhurn P, Bing C, Wood IS. Adipose tissue and adipokines--energy regulation from the human perspective. *J Nutr.* 2006 Jul;136(7 Suppl):1935S-1939S.
>
> E) Maachi M, Pieroni L, Bruckert E, Jardel C, Fellahi S, Hainque B, Capeau J, Bastard JP. Systemic low-grade inflammation is related to both circulating and adipose tissue TNFalpha, leptin and IL-6 levels in obese women. *Int J Obes Relat Metab Disord.* 2004 Aug;28(8):993-7.
>
> F) Ferrier KE, Nestel P, Taylor A, Drew BG, Kingwell BA. Diet but not aerobic exercise training reduces skeletal muscle TNF-alpha in overweight humans. *Diabetologia.* 2004 Mar 26 [Epub ahead of print]
>
> G) Devaraj S, O'Keefe G, Jialal I. Defining the proinflammatory phenotype using high sensitive C-reactive protein levels as the biomarker. *J Clin Endocrinol Metab.* 2005 Aug;90(8):4549-54. Epub 2005 May 17.
>
> H) Visser M, Bouter LM, McQuillan GM, Wener MH, Harris TB. Elevated C-reactive protein levels in overweight and obese

adults. *JAMA.* 1999 Dec 8;282(22):2131-5

I) Saijo Y, Kiyota N, Kawasaki Y, Miyazaki Y, Kashimura J, Fukuda M, Kishi R. Relationship between C-reactive protein and visceral adipose tissue in healthy Japanese subjects. *Diabetes Obes Metab.* 2004 Jul;6(4):249-58.

J) Trayhurn P. Endocrine and signaling role of adipose tissue: new perspectives on fat. *Acta Physiol Scand.* 2005 Aug;184(4):285-93.

K) Shamsuzzaman AS, Winnicki M, Wolk R, Svatikova A, Phillips BG, Davison DE, Berger PB, Somers VK. Independent association between plasma leptin and C-reactive protein in healthy humans. Circulation. 2004 May 11;109(18):2181-5. Epub 2004 Apr 26.

L) Bullo M, Garcia-Lorda P, Megias I, Salas-Salvado J. Systemic inflammation, adipose tissue tumor necrosis factor, and leptin expression. *Obes Res.* 2003 Apr;11(4):525-31.

M) Ble A, Windham BG, Bandinelli S, Taub DD, Volpato S, Bartali B, Tracy RP, Guralnik JM, Ferrucci L. Relation of Plasma Leptin to C-Reactive Protein in Older Adults (from the Invecchiare nel Chianti Study). *Am J Cardiol.* 2005 Oct 1;96(7):991-5.

N) Roubenoff R, Parise H, Payette HA, Abad LW, D'Agostino R, Jacques PF, Wilson PW, Dinarello CA, Harris TB. Cytokines, insulin-like growth factor 1, sarcopenia, and mortality in very old community-dwelling men and women: the Framingham Heart Study. *Am J Med.* 2003 Oct 15;115(6):429-35.

Leptin problems are not only a top risk factor for heart disease, these problems cause heart disease in numerous different ways, often simultaneously.

Researchers demonstrate that elevated leptin is a primary risk factor for a first heart attack in men.

Thogersen AM, Soderberg S, Jansson JH, Dahlen G, Boman K, Nilsson TK, Lindahl B, Weinehall L, Stenlund H, Lundberg V, Johnson O, Ahren B, Hallmans G. Interactions between fibrinolysis, lipoproteins and leptin related to a first myocardial infarction. *Eur J Cardiovasc Prev Rehabil.* 2004 Feb;11(1):33-40.

Researchers show that leptin problems directly elevate blood pressure.

A) Tsuda K, Nishio I. Leptin and membrane fluidity of erythrocytes in essential hypertension: an electron paramagnetic resonance investigation. *Am J Hypertens.* 2004 Apr;17(4):375-9.

B) Pantanetti P, Garrapa GG, Mantero F, Boscaro M, Faloia E, Venarucci D. Adipose tissue as an endocrine organ? A review of recent data related to cardiovascular complications of endocrine dysfunctions. *Clin Exp Hypertens.* 2004 May;26(4):387-98.

C) Martins D, Tareen N, Pan D, Norris K. The relationship between body mass index, blood pressure and pulse rate among normotensive and hypertensive participants in the third National Health and Nutrition Examination Survey (NHANES). *Cell Mol Biol (Noisy-le-grand).* 2003 Dec;49(8):1305-9.

Several studies show that one reason for leptin-driven elevated blood pressure is kidney damage. Abdominal obesity is consistent with the increased inflammation that damages the kidneys.

A) Bosma RJ, Krikken JA, Homan van der Heide JJ, de Jong PE, Navis GJ. Obesity and renal hemodynamics. *Contrib Nephrol.* 2006;151:184-202.

B) Rutkowski P, Klassen A, Sebekova K, Bahner U, Heidland A. Renal disease in obesity: the need for greater attention. *J Ren Nutr.* 2006 Jul;16(3):216-23.

C) Beltowski J, Wojcicka G, Marciniak A, Jamroz A. Oxidative stress, nitric oxide production, and renal sodium handling in leptin-induced hypertension. *Life Sci.* 2004 Apr 30;74(24):2987-3000.

Researchers explain how normal leptin levels help regulate cardiovascular function and that elevated leptin levels are a direct risk factor for high cholesterol, high blood pressure, and heart disease.

A) Ren J. Leptin and hyperleptinemia - from friend to foe for cardiovascular function. J Endocrinol. 2004 Apr;181(1):1-10.

B) Rahmouni K, Haynes WG. Leptin and the cardiovascular system. Recent Prog Horm Res. 2004;59:225-44.

Researchers confirm that leptin problems are a key risk factor for cardiovascular health, including the risk for high cholesterol and high blood pressure.

Zamboni M, Zoico E, Fantin F, Panourgia MP, Di Francesco V, Tosoni P, Solerte B, Vettor R, Bosello O. Relation between leptin and the metabolic syndrome in elderly women.*J Gerontol A Biol Sci Med Sci.* 2004 Apr;59(4):396-400.

Researchers make a major discovery, finding that cholesterol synthesis is, in part, regulated by leptin entering the brain properly. Leptin problems, reflected by eating too much or too little, thus directly elevate cholesterol. This is the first time a specific mechanism of excessive cholesterol synthesis due to brain function has been identified.

Vanpatten S, Karkanias GB, Rossetti L, Cohen DE. Intracerebroventricular leptin regulates hepatic cholesterol metabolism. *Biochem J.* 2004 Apr 15;379(Pt 2):229-33.

Researchers find that waist circumference is the most predictive physical measurement relating to coronary artery disease in overweight premenopausal women and that leptin levels are directly elevated in proportion to waist measurement.

Lofgren I, Herron K, Zern T, West K, Patalay M, Shachter NS, Koo SI, Fernandez ML. Waist circumference is a better predictor than body mass index of coronary heart disease risk in overweight premenopausal women. *J Nutr.* 2004 May;134(5):1071-6.

Researchers outline numerous substances coming from fat cells, including leptin, that directly interact with and regulate the cardiovascular system. Their research demonstrates an elaborate communication network between fat cells and blood vessels.

Fruhbeck G. The Adipose Tissue as a Source of Vasoactive Factors. *Curr Med Chem Cardiovasc Hematol Agents.* 2004 Jul;2(3):197-208.

Researchers show for the first time that leptin is made by heart cells and heart cells receive leptin messages. This means the heart can act independently (and intelligently) to make and regulate its own energy production via proper leptin function.

It also means that leptin problems are likely to directly interfere with normal heart energy production. This is a major finding.

Purdham DM, Zou MX, Rajapurohitam V, Karmazyn M. The Rat Heart is a Site of Leptin Production and Action. Am J Physiol Heart Circ Physiol. 2004 Jul 29

Researchers show that leptin problems are a prime risk for all factors of the metabolic syndrome (high cholesterol, high blood pressure, insulin resistance, and weight gain) that is reflective of heart disease risk.

Li M, Wu CY, Zhan ZW, Li XG, Zhang K, Xiang HD. Leptin and clustering of the components of risk factors for metabolic syndrome *Zhonghua Yu Fang Yi Xue Za Zhi*. 2004 Jul;38(4):226-30.

Researchers show that leptin problems are a key risk factor for a first stroke in men.

Soderberg S, Stegmayr B, Stenlund H, Sjostrom LG, Agren A, Johansson L, Weinehall L, Olsson T. Leptin, but not adiponectin, predicts stroke in males. *J Intern Med.* 2004 Aug;256(2):128-36.

Leptin resistance and abdominal obesity are direct risk factors for stroke.

Kurukulasuriya LR, Govindarajan G, Sowers J. Stroke prevention in diabetes and obesity. *Expert Rev Cardiovasc Ther.* 2006 Jul;4(4):487-502.

Leptin resistance increases platelet activation, a stickiness in the blood that may promote a clot that causes stroke.

Wallaschofski H, Kobsar A, Sokolova O, Eigenthaler M, Lohmann T. Co-activation of platelets by prolactin or leptin--pathophysiological findings and clinical implications. *Horm Metab Res.* 2004 Jan;36(1):1-6.

In some cases, high leptin-driven inflammation may damage or destroy platelets.

Zhan M, Zhao H, Yang R, Han ZC. Serum leptin levels in patients with idiopathic thrombocytopenic purpura. *Eur J Haematol.* 2004 May;72(5):348-52.

High leptin induces oxidative stress leading to clogged arteries.

Beltowski J, Wojcicka G, Jamroz A. Leptin decreases plasma para-oxonase 1 (PON1) activity and induces oxidative stress: the possible novel mechanism for proatherogenic effect of chronic hyperlepti-nemia. *Atherosclerosis.* 2003 Sep;170(1):21-9.

Leptin problems promote general clogging of arteries by provoking fat to accumulate in vascular smooth muscle.

Davies JD, Carpenter KL, Challis IR, Figg NL, McNair R, Proud-foot D, Weissberg PL, Shanahan CM. Adipocytic differentiation and liver x receptor pathways regulate the accumulation of triacylglycer-ols in human vascular smooth muscle cells. *J Biol Chem.* 2005 Feb 4;280(5):3911-9. Epub 2004 Nov 16.

Even modest weight loss reduces heart disease risk.

Valsamakis G, McTernan Pg P, Chetty R, Al Daghri N, Field A, Hanif W, Barnett Ah A, Kumar S. Modest weight loss and reduction in waist circumference after medical treatment are associated with favorable changes in serum adipocytokines. *Metabolism.* 2004 Apr;53(4):430-4.

Sustained modest weight loss reduces cardiovascular risk, even when the goal weight is not yet reached.

Pasanisi F, Contaldo F, de Simone G, Mancini M. Benefits of sus-tained moderate weight loss in obesity. *Nutr Metab Cardiovasc Dis.* 2001 Dec;11(6):401-6.

THE FIVE RULES

Eating in harmony with leptin is the key to successful weight loss and returning leptin to more normal function, which in turn reduces health risks.

Rule 1 – Never eat after dinner

A) Proper leptin release over a 24-hour period is based on meal timing. Schoeller DA, Cella LK, Sinha MK, Caro JF. Entrain-ment of the diurnal rhythm of plasma leptin to meal timing. J Clin Invest. 1997 Oct 1;100(7):1882-7.

B) Leptin 24-hour rhythm, blunted in obesity. Radic R, Nikolic V, Karner I, Kosovic P, Kurbel S, Selthofer R, Curkovic M. Circadian rhythm of blood leptin level in obese and non-obese people. *Coll Antropol.* 2003 Dec;27(2):555-61.

C) Disrupted leptin 24-hour rhythm disturbs nighttime repair, blunting growth hormone. Heptulla R, Smitten A, Teague B, Tamborlane WV, Ma YZ, Caprio S. Temporal patterns of circulating leptin levels in lean and obese adolescents: relationships to insulin, growth hormone, and free fatty acids rhythmicity. *J Clin Endocrinol Metab*. 2001 Jan;86(1):90-6.

D) Leptin problems cause sleep apnea. Patel SR, Palmer LJ, Larkin EK, Jenny NS, White DP, Redline S. Relationship between obstructive sleep apnea and diurnal leptin rhythms. *Sleep*. 2004 Mar 15;27(2):235-9.

E) Problems in the 24-hour leptin pattern induce excess food intake. Chin-Chance C, Polonsky KS, Schoeller DA. Twenty-four-hour leptin levels respond to cumulative short-term energy imbalance and predict subsequent intake. *J Clin Endocrinol Metab*. 2000 Aug;85(8):2685-91.

F) There is also a leptin-insulin rhythm in response to a meal. Frequent smaller meals increase insulin, stress general leptin function, and disturb the 24-hour leptin pattern. (see Rule 2). Fogteloo AJ, Pijl H, Roelfsema F, Frolich M, Meinders AE. Impact of meal timing and frequency on the twenty-four-hour leptin rhythm. *Horm Res*. 2004;62(2):71-8. Epub 2004 Jun 21.

Rule 2 – Eat three meals a day – do not snack

A) Leptin rises in response to any meal. Elimam A, Marcus C. Meal timing, fasting and glucocorticoids interplay in serum leptin concentrations and diurnal profile. *Eur J Endocrinol*. 2002 Aug;147(2):181-8.

B) Normal leptin release following the meal turns off pancreatic insulin production, a response that is blunted in leptin resistance (causing overeating). Seufert J. Leptin effects on pancreatic beta-cell gene expression and function. *Diabetes*. 2004 Feb;53 Suppl 1:S152-8.

C) Normal leptin release following the meal turns off pancreatic insulin production, a response that is blunted in leptin resistance (causing overeating). Heini AF, Lara-Castro C, Kirk KA, Considine RV, Caro JF, Weinsier RL. Association of leptin and hunger-satiety ratings in obese women. Int J Obes Relat Metab Disord. 1998 Nov;22(11):1084-7.

D) Learned pancreatic "addictive" insulin response. Raben A,

Astrup A. Leptin is influenced both by predisposition to obesity and diet composition. *Int J Obes Relat Metab Disord*. 2000 Apr;24(4):450-9.

E) Increasing the amount of time between meals improves brain function and reduces brain susceptibility to age-associated brain damage, independent of the total calories eaten. Mattson MP, Duan W, Guo Z. Meal size and frequency affect neuronal plasticity and vulnerability to disease: cellular and molecular mechanisms. *J Neurochem*. 2003 Feb;84(3):417-31.

F) Fasting between meals (no snacking) reduces cardiovascular disease and improves brain function, in part by lessening oxidative damage and improving cellular stress tolerance. Mattson MP, Wan R. Beneficial effects of intermittent fasting and caloric restriction on the cardiovascular and cerebrovascular systems. *J Nutr Biochem*. 2005 Mar;16(3):129-37.

Rule 3 – Do not eat large meals

A) Large meals are a fast way to induce leptin problems. Van Aggel-Leijssen DP, van Baak MA, Tenenbaum R, Campfield LA, Saris WH. Regulation of average 24h human plasma leptin level; the influence of exercise and physiological changes in energy balance. *Int J Obes Relat Metab Disord*. 1999 Feb;23(2):151-8.

B) Large portions cause people to eat more and directly induce obesity. Rolls,BJ, Morri,ER and Roe LS Portion size of food affects energy intake in normal-weight and overweight men and women *Am J Clin Nutr* 2002;76:1207–13.

C) Overweight people have great difficulty with digestive signals that properly communicate a *full* signal to the brain, predisposing them to further overeating at meals. Schwartz GJ. Biology of eating behavior in obesity. *Obes Res*. 2004 Nov;12 Suppl 2:102S-6S.

D) Studies with twins show that overeating fuels leptin-related gene weaknesses, causing leptin problems and obesity. Ukkola O, Bouchard C. Role of candidate genes in the responses to long-term overfeeding: review of findings. *Obes Rev*. 2004 Feb;5(1):3-12.

E) Eating too much damages the brain, leading to cognitive decline in older age. Reduced food intake preserves and enhances brain function. Mattson MP. Neuroprotective signaling and the aging brain: take away my food and let me run. *Brain Res.* 2000 Dec 15;886(1-2):47-53.

F) Binge eating flares leptin problems. Taylor AE, Hubbard J, Anderson EJ. Impact of binge eating on metabolic and leptin dynamics in normal young women. J Clin Endocrinol Metab. 1999 Feb;84(2):428-34.

G) Overfeeding induces lipotoxicity. Unger RH. Longevity, lipotoxicity and leptin: the adipocyte defense against feasting and famine. *Biochimie.* 2005 Jan;87(1):57-64.

H) Leptin resistance induces overeating, high levels of insulin, and inappropriate desire for increased food intake due to abnormal dopamine function. Lustig RH. Childhood obesity: behavioral aberration or biochemical drive? Reinterpreting the First Law of Thermodynamics. *Nat Clin Pract Endocrinol Metab.* 2006 Aug;2(8):447-58.

I) Even moderate physical activity helps restore normal leptin appetite *full* signals in obese women. Tsofliou F, Pitsiladis YP, Malkova D, Wallace AM, Lean ME. Moderate physical activity permits acute coupling between serum leptin and appetite-satiety measures in obese women. Int J Obes Relat Metab Disord. 2003 Nov;27(11):1332-9.

Rule 4 – Eat a breakfast containing protein

A) Activation of liver metabolism may be as high as 30% for 12 hours following a high-protein meal. Guyton A. Specific dynamic action of protein. Textbook of Medical Physiology WB Saunders Company 1991:793-4.

B) A high-protein meal increased metabolic activity by 17% in normal weight women, compared to a high fat or high carbohydrate meal. Raben A, Agerholm-Larsen L, Flint A, Holst JJ, Astrup A. Meals with similar energy densities but rich in protein, fat, carbohydrate, or alcohol have different effects on energy expenditure and substrate metabolism but not on appetite and energy intake. *J Clin Nutr.* 2003 Jan;77(1):91-100.

C) Under carefully monitored laboratory conditions, a high-protein breakfast in men suppressed hunger over a 24-hour period compared to a high-carbohydrate or high-fat breakfast. Stubbs RJ, van Wyk MC, Johnstone AM, Harbron CG. Breakfasts high in protein, fat or carbohydrate: effect on within-day appetite and energy balance. *Eur J Clin Nutr.* 1996 Jul;50(7):409-17.

D) Leptin patterns are more stable later in the day from higher protein intake. Polson DA, Thompson MP. Macronutrient composition of the diet differentially affects leptin and adiponutrin mRNA expression in response to meal feeding. *J Nutr Biochem.* 2004 Apr;15(4):242-6.

E) Higher protein helps stabilization of blood sugar. Koutsari C, Karpe F, Humphreys SM, Frayn KN, Hardman AE. Plasma leptin is influenced by diet composition and exercise. *Int J Obes Relat Metab Disord.* 2003 Aug;27(8):901-6.

F) Moderate calorie restriction in combination with a higher protein diet reduces leptin and insulin problems in overweight premenopausl women. Lofgren IE, Herron KL, West KL, Zern TL, Brownbill RA, Ilich JZ, Koo SI, Fernandez ML. Weight loss favorably modifies anthropometrics and reverses the metabolic syndrome in premenopausal women. *J Am Coll Nutr.* 2005 Dec;24(6):486-93.

G) Daily protein intake at thirty percent of calories reduces leptin, lowers appetite, and facilitates weight loss compared to an intake of fifteen percent protein and higher carbohydrates. Weigle DS, Breen PA, Matthys CC, Callahan HS, Meeuws KE, Burden VR, Purnell JQ. A high-protein diet induces sustained reductions in appetite, ad libitum caloric intake, and body weight despite compensatory changes in diurnal plasma leptin and ghrelin concentrations. *Am J Clin Nutr.* 2005 Jul;82(1):41-8.

H) Higher protein intake helps prevent weight gain following weight loss. Westerterp-Plantenga MS, Lejeune MP, Nijs I, van Ooijen M, Kovacs EM. High protein intake sustains weight maintenance after body weight loss in humans. *Int J Obes Relat Metab Disord.* 2004 Jan;28(1):57-64.

I) Higher protein helps stabilization of blood sugar. Koutsari C, Karpe F, Humphreys SM, Frayn KN, Hardman AE. Plasma leptin is influenced by diet composition and exercise. *Int J Obes Relat Metab Disord.* 2003 Aug;27(8):901-6.

J) Dietary proteins, such as whey protein, enhance the *full* feeling more effectively than glucose. Bowen J, Noakes M, Trenerry C, Clifton PM. Energy intake, ghrelin, and cholecystokinin after different carbohydrate and protein preloads in overweight men. *J Clin Endocrinol Metab.* 2006 Apr;91(4):1477-83. Epub

2006 Jan 24.

K) A whey-protein breakfast in overweight men significantly reduces post-meal glucose levels and reduces the amount of food freely eaten at lunch. Bowen J, Noakes M, Clifton P, Jenkins A, Batterham M. Acute effect of dietary proteins on appetite, energy intake and glycemic response in overweight men. *Asia Pac J Clin Nutr.* 2004;13(Suppl):S64.

L) A breakfast containing eggs produced a *full* feeling much more effectively than a similar-calorie bagel breakfast, resulting in significantly less eating later in the morning. Vander Wal JS, Marth JM, Khosla P, Jen KL, Dhurandhar NV. Short-term effect of eggs on satiety in overweight and obese subjects. *J Am Coll Nutr.* 2005 Dec;24(6):510-5.

M) In normal-weight and overweight children, the higher the carbohydrate content of the breakfast, the greater the amount of food eaten at lunch. Warren JM, Henry CJ, Simonite V. Low glycemic index breakfasts and reduced food intake in preadolescent children. *Pediatrics.* 2003 Nov;112(5):e414.

Rule 5 – Reduce the amount of carbohydrate eaten

A) The higher the carbohydrate intake, the greater the leptin activation. Yannakoulia M, Yiannakouris N, Bluher S, Matalas AL, Klimis-Zacas D, Mantzoros CS Body fat mass and macronutrient intake in relation to circulating soluble leptin receptor, free leptin index, adiponectin, and resistin concentrations in healthy humans. *J Clin Endocrinol Metab.* 2003 Apr;88(4):1730-6.

B) As obesity develops, carbohydrate cravings are increased, provoking further weight gain and leptin disturbance. Wang J, Akabayashi A, Dourmashkin J, Yu HJ, Alexander JT, Chae HJ, Leibowitz SF. Neuropeptide Y in relation to carbohydrate intake, corticosterone and dietary obesity. (rat study) Brain Res. 1998 Aug 17;802(1-2):75-88.

C) Overweight premenopausal women who reduced carbohydrate intake, total calories, and increased exercise reduced disease-provoking small LDL particles by 26%. Lofgren I, Zern T, Herron K, West K, Sharman MJ, Volek JS, Shachter NS, Koo SI, Fernandez ML. Weight loss associated with reduced intake of carbohydrate reduces the atherogenicity of LDL in premenopausal women. *Metabolism.* 2005 Sep;54(9):1133-41.

D) Carbohydrate restriction can reduce abdominal fat by 20% in overweight men and improve cholesterol function, reducing the risk for cardiovascular disease. Wood RJ, Volek JS, Liu Y, Shachter NS, Contois JH, Fernandez ML. Carbohydrate restriction alters lipoprotein metabolism by modifying VLDL, LDL, and HDL subfraction distribution and size in overweight men. *J Nutr.* 2006 Feb;136(2):384-9.

E) A meal containing 70% sugar induces an abnormal five-fold increased release of insulin compared to a meal that is 70% protein, which does not stimulate leptin release (rat study). Polson DA, Thompson MP. Macronutrient composition of the diet differentially affects leptin and adiponutrin mRNA expression in response to meal feeding. *J Nutr Biochem.* 2004 Apr;15(4):242-6.

F) Fructose-sweetened beverages fool the brain into calorie over-consumption. Bray GA, Nielsen SJ, Popkin BM. Consumption of high-fructose corn syrup in beverages may play a role in the epidemic of obesity. *Am J Clin Nutr.* 2004 Apr;79(4):537-43

G) High-fructose corn syrup induces greater leptin resistance than does excessive fat intake (neither is good). Huang BW, Chiang MT, Yao HT, Chiang W. The effect of high-fat and high-fructose diets on glucose tolerance and plasma lipid and leptin levels in rats. *Diabetes Obes Metab.* 2004 Mar;6(2):120-6

H) Higher glycemic index eating causes increased insulin resistance. Brynes AE, Mark Edwards C, Ghatei MA, Dornhorst A, Morgan LM, Bloom SR, Frost GS. A randomised four-intervention crossover study investigating the effect of carbohydrates on daytime profiles of insulin, glucose, non-esterified fatty acids and triacylglycerols in middle-aged men. *Br J Nutr.* 2003 Feb;89(2):207-18.

A FEW POINTS ABOUT DIET

Cholesterol from eggs is not related to cardiovascular disease.

A) McNamara DJ. The impact of egg limitations on coronary heart disease risk: do the numbers add up? Comment in: J Am Coll Nutr. 2001 Feb;20(1):93-4. *J Am Coll Nutr.* 2000 Oct;19(5 Suppl):540S-548S.

B) Kritchevsky SB, Kritchevsky D. Egg consumption and coronary heart disease: an epidemiologic overview. *J Am Coll Nutr.*

2000 Oct;19(5 Suppl):549S-555S.

C) Milk-fat intake is negatively associated with heart disease and leptin levels. Warensjo E, Jansson JH, Berglund L, Boman K, Ahren B, Weinehall L, Lindahl B, Hallmans G, Vessby B. Estimated intake of milk fat is negatively associated with cardiovascular risk factors and does not increase the risk of a first acute myocardial infarction. A prospective case-control study. *Br J Nutr.* 2004 Apr;91(4):635-42.

D) Antioxidants and caffeine are synergistic in enhancing weight-loss function. Zheng G, Sayama K, Okubo T, Juneja LR, Oguni I. Anti-obesity effects of three major components of green tea, catechins, caffeine and theanine, in mice. *In Vivo.* 2004 Jan-Feb;18(1):55-62.

E) Too much caffeine may suppress leptin and cause increased weight regain following a starvation diet. Kovacs EM, Lejeune MP, Nijs I, Westerterp-Plantenga MS. Effects of green tea on weight maintenance after body-weight loss. *Br J Nutr.* 2004 Mar;91(3):431-7.

F) Higher omega 3 in the diet results in less arthritis due to reduced inflammation. Hagfors L, Nilsson I, Skoldstam L, Johansson G. Fat intake and composition of fatty acids in serum phospholipids in a randomized, controlled, Mediterranean dietary intervention study on patients with rheumatoid arthritis. *Nutr Metab (Lond).* 2005 Oct 10;2(1):26 [Epub ahead of print]

INDEX